Pearls
of
Birth

Wisdom

Pearls of Birth Wisdom.
Published by Castenetto & Co 2020.
©Tessa Venuti Sanderson

Tessa Venuti Sanderson has asserted her moral right to be identified as the author of this work in accordance with the Copyright, Designs and Patent Act of 1988.

ISBN 978-0-9933751-8-7

British Library Cataloguing-in-Publication Data.
A catalogue record for this book is available from the British Library.

Editor and proofread by Davene Wasser
Cover and internal layout Emy Farella
Printed and bound by KPD.

www.pearlsofbirthwisdom.com

Disclaimer: Please note that this book provides general information about pregnancy, labour and birth and does not constitute medical advice for individuals. Please consult your own healthcare providers when making decisions that may affect your health or that of your baby. If you need further support or advice please use the following resources: birthrights.org.uk, maternityaction. org.uk (employment and working rights), aims.org.uk (promoting normal birth, rights and choice; has helpline), and whiteribbonalliance.org (see their Respectful Maternity Care Charter).

For Mum, Dad and Jojo.

Thank you to the parents who so generously shared their stories with us, and the midwives and other health professionals who cared for them.

About the author

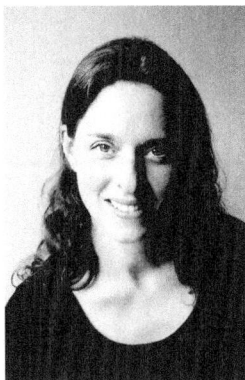

Tessa Venuti Sanderson is an experienced Pregnancy Yoga teacher who lives in Berkshire, UK, with her partner and two children. She has a PhD in Medical Sociology and was a post-doctoral researcher until her second maternity leave. She has an MSc in Exercise, Nutrition and Public Health and has more than 20 academic papers related to patient wellbeing and prioritising outcomes important to patients.

She is an active member of the Maternity Voices Forum at the Royal Berkshire Hospital for four years and has contributed to the development of the new Patient Portal enabling easier access to records through smartphones.

As well writing about pregnancy and birth for a number of publications, including Juno, Mother & Baby and Green Parent magazines, and her own Pregnancy and Birth Colouring Book, Tessa has written a series of children's books about anatomy and puberty: Ruby Luna's Curious Journey, Ruby Luna's Moontime and Dante Leon's Curious Journey.

Contents

List of boxes with practices

Foreword

The divine irony of reading books on birth is that the very act of reading takes us away from the fierce living experience of birth. An experience that confronted us on a daily basis before both birth and we became industrialised.

What truly can prepare us for an experience as raw and personal and physical as birth? Birth is a verb before it is a noun: a moving, living, embodied experience that like a river flows always downwards but like many rivers takes turns and unexpected crescendos according to the weather and the terrain. The birth process itself follows a chartered course, but along that course the experience is always unique.

Birth is a bodily not a mental experience, and Tessa elegantly weaves her expertise in body awareness and embodied practices with the stories of many women who have shared their intimate birth journeys with us. It is an ancient practice, this sharing of personal stories, one that brings us as close to participation as the leaves of a book can bring. Tessa brings birth back to where it belongs: the body, and the exercises, practices and resources are awakening and empowering to women undertaking parenthood and the challenges of life beyond.

Most potently, Tessa offers pearls, Pearls of Wisdom, to orient us to the reality that our female bodies know how to birth - given appropriate safety. Birth is as intrinsic as eating and sleeping, as pooping and peeing. Yet none of these processes work efficiently in a context of fear. The Pearls she offers are beads of safety, stars of safe passage to navigate through the often-stormy seas of birth, simply explained and supported by current breakthroughs in the fields of neuroscience and the understanding of trauma and its resolution.

If you need a companion for your birth, take Tessa with you. Doula, mentor, mother, sister, guide to your inner wisdom, the wisdom of the best guide you will have: your own sweet, unique, exquisitely intelligent body.

Welcome home!

Giselle Genillard

L'Arche, 14 July 2020
Director of SOS Internationale, providing Somatic Experiencing training, and Midwife.

Introduction

My journey into meditation and other aspects of yoga started long before my first pregnancy. When I took my first meditation class, I did not realise how much the practice would prepare me for birth one day. Over the years of teaching pregnancy yoga, I have witnessed the amazing support that mindfulness and movement can bring to the birth journey. I have taught over a thousand women and I never get tired of seeing the transformation from anxious to calmly anticipatory.

As I write this, my daughters are 9 and 7. It feels like only yesterday that I was pregnant. My children inspire me every day to make the greatest impact that I can in this lifetime for women and girls. I've felt called to collate these birth stories because the birth of a child is a rite of passage – a series of events that will always stay with you. If it's a 'good' birth, then it will remind you how awesome you are and how awesome your body is. If it's a challenging or traumatic birth, then it may be like a heavy weight or a feeling like your chest collapsing in, when it's not packed away in a box inside your head. I'm not mincing my words here – you can have a big impact on the birth of your baby, but it takes preparation. The more you can face the journey head on, however daunting that may feel, the more prepared you can be. This is not a journey like any other, and however you come out the other side, you will be forever changed. It is the heroine's journey.

When I hold Mother Blessings for expectant mums, we often make a birthing necklace. The friends and family members will bring a bead that is symbolic in some way of pregnancy, birth or parenting. We pass the thread around the circle and the very different beads are added one by one. The necklaces are often not neat and definitely not symmetrical, but these necklaces are a thing of great beauty. Each necklace is unique, holding both memories and hopefulness about the future. In this way, the necklace becomes a symbol of the birthing process.

This book focuses on the inner journey that you can take to make this rite of passage an empowering one. You will hear three different voices in this book: the birth stories are like the beads on a necklace, my narrative as a pregnancy yoga teacher is the thread, and the exercises and reflections are the beads you can add yourself. You can add many beads or none at all, but this is a time when more is definitely better.

I hope you will read the birth stories with an open heart. They have been generously shared by parents from my classes or birth preparation workshops and have not been selected because they are 'perfect' examples of how to 'do' birth, but because they are real and positive for the storyteller. The stories are sacred because they tell of the entrance of a human being into the world.

Each time I receive a birth story I feel privileged and touched to have an insight into the journey that the parents and child have taken. You may see yourself in the hopes and expectations of some stories, but not find common ground in others. The stories show the diversity of how the birth journey unfolds and how wisdom can grow from experience. By sharing these experiences, my hope is that even if this is your first baby, you can understand what will support *you* in making this journey safely and unlocking the gifts of the birth initiation.

The cocoon of safety

What is coming is the most important line of the whole book: for birth to be experienced and remembered as a positive journey, you need to feel safe. **For birth to be experienced and remembered as a positive journey, you need to feel safe.** Take a deep breath and really let that sink in.

Feeling safe is a basic human right. To enjoy making love, we need to feel safe. It's much easier to poo if you feel safe! We want our children to grow up in safety. For birth to unfold smoothly we need to feel safe. Achieving a feeling of safety happens on many levels: in our minds, bodies and environment. Throughout our lives as individuals we may have received different messages about how to be safe, and in this book, we will look at different aspects that may affect the birthing journey. They will either affect it subconsciously or consciously. The choice is yours, but I would rather know what I'm dealing with and take steps to make the journey easier when I can.

I recognise that not everyone starts from a feeling of safety in their everyday lives, but I hope the content of this book will support ways for you to experience what it is to be safe before the birth of your baby.

There is no judgement on how your baby is born: from freebirthing (no health professionals in attendance) to elective caesarean birth, that is from no intervention to a high level of intervention, these are all valid ways that babies make their way into the world. Feeling safe is not only possible, but critical throughout the whole spectrum and you can be a part of decision-making in every scenario. What I want to offer you is a chance to take ownership of the birth journey and of your body, and that of your baby's (held tenderly until your child is old enough to take ownership themselves). This is what ultimately makes you feel safe and empowered.

What I see happen in my classes regularly, is a realisation of what the female body is capable of and a reclaiming of sovereignty. Sometimes this means that a woman will change her assumption that she will be on the delivery suite with all options for pain relief on hand, to a recognition that a homebirth is what would make her feel most safe. Or it may mean that she declines routine vaginal examinations or sweeps. Or that she pushes for an elective caesarean because that is what feels most safe for her at the time. I want you to remember the birth of your baby as a time when you were listened to and respected. While there are a number of factors outside of your control, there is a lot that you can do.

Let's see how to create this cocoon of safety within ourselves and our environments.

A note to the reader

Each chapter is structured as follows: introduction to the pearl of wisdom, birth stories, exercises, reflections and resources. The only selection criteria for the birth stories is that the parent writing it views it as a positive birth story. They have not been edited to show only the positive parts because I want to share the reality of the journey so you can learn from all of these parents' experiences.

I have selected a few key exercises from my pregnancy yoga classes and birth preparation workshops to share with you. You'll find these as a way to elaborate on something a woman touched on in her birthing story (see boxes).

The reflection section in each chapter is designed to make you think deeply and so may trigger challenging feelings and uncomfortable thoughts. Sometimes it will be enough that you have felt the emotions that arise and understood the effect of the question on you, but other times you may need support. Please share your reflections in the **Community of Pearls Facebook group** (or if you identify that greater support is needed, talk to your midwife or self-refer to Talking Therapies).

The reflections are about potentially big and deep emotions, and it may be that you could not do justice to them all during one pregnancy! Please do not be overwhelmed by the resources and reflections but focus on where you feel most called during this inner journey. I recommend keeping a journal or downloading the free **Pearls of Wisdom journal booklet**, which contains all the questions in one place with space to record your reflections. This and other free downloads mentioned in the text are available at **www.pearlsofbirthwisdom.com/downloads.**

If you are a birth professional, I invite you to also answer the questions in the Reflection sections as a way to engage more deeply with the content. If you already have children, you might reflect back on your decisions previously and what you would change for another pregnancy. If you do not have children, I wonder if you can imagine how you would feel if you were carrying a child and were faced with a whole world of decisions to be made.

Over the years I have amassed a big collection of books, articles and helpful internet material. I share some relevant resources at the end of each chapter to enable further reading if you want to go deeper into the topic. Some of the topics raised are big ones, and we can only scratch the surface in this book. If you choose to make use of these resources, perhaps focus on one or two topics that seem most pertinent to your pregnancy or upcoming birth. All of the websites mentioned in the resources, plus a list of recommended podcasts, can be found at **www.pearlsofbirthwisdom.com/downloads** so you can easily find the right content for you.

Disclaimer: the content in this book does not replace medical advice but is aimed to get the reader to think critically about what is being offered during antenatal, birth and postnatal care. All of the pearls are relevant to those with a normal, healthy pregnancy as well as to those with complications.

Pearl 1
Soothing

*A soothing atmosphere allows
the body to soften and relax.
Then the body can be present
and ready for whatever comes.*

Imagine that you feel calm and take a deep breath. Your eyes are closed, and you can hear soothing music in the background. You know that if you open your eyes you will see fairy lights giving just enough light for you to move around the room. You can feel your birth partner's hand on your shoulder giving you quiet reassurance, and you are resting on soft pillows. You feel gently focused, conserving your energy for what is to come: the birth of your baby.

Our nervous system has evolved to be in one of two states: on alert, with the sympathetic nervous system priming us to fight, run or freeze; OR calm, with the parasympathetic nervous system allowing the body to rest and digest (and give birth). Our culture of being busy, with endless stimulation, means that we are often stressed and get used to adrenalin circulating. However, our body evolved only to handle short bursts of adrenalin and if we are chronically stressed, we feel the effects with indigestion, poor sleep and a compromised immune system.

The part of the brain (the reptilian, or "old", brain) that controls birth is the same as for digestion. It is not actively under our control. If we want to digest our breakfast, we do not sit there and think "now food, move from the stomach into the intestines, peristalsis move that bolus of food along...": it is done without our conscious control. Birth is similar because we cannot control how quickly our cervix effaces or dilates; or when the contractions start, how often they come or how long they last.

What we *can* influence a lot of the time, is how safe we feel and give our nervous system the best chance of being in the parasympathetic state. There are many things that can influence your sense of safety. These will be different for everyone – you will need to do some reflection in order to create your unique cocoon of safety. There are many ways of supporting your nervous system directly, including meditation, relaxation tracks, breathing techniques and calming movement like yoga. Throughout the book, we will explore many of these different factors.

Following is a mother's story about her first birthing.

ANNA'S BIRTHING STORY

(homebirth, waterbirth)

Anna is a friendly and witty professional, who asked lots of questions in the pregnancy yoga classes and the birth preparation workshop. I could see she prepares for everything that she does in life!

Rory's birth:

As this was my first pregnancy and I was considered low risk, when I had my midwife appointments, I was informed I was eligible to give birth in the midwife-led unit at the Royal Berkshire Hospital. The option of having a homebirth was not discussed. It was not until my husband Matt and I attended an NCT [National Childbirth Trust] course that the option of homebirth was discussed in more detail and we started thinking about it as an option that could work for us. Further, when we attended Tessa's birth preparation workshop and we discussed the importance of feeling calm and safe in your environment, I thought I would feel a lot more relaxed and comfortable in my own home than in hospital.

I was also keen on having a water birth and aware that this may not work out if I went into hospital and all the birth pools were being used at that time. Therefore, at about 37–38 weeks pregnant (cutting it pretty fine!) I asked to be transferred to the care of the homebirth midwife team (who were great). I had a friend who had attempted to have a homebirth (unfortunately it did not work out for her) who had told me she wished she had used a doula to support her birth and this got me started on considering using a doula. I did not have much idea of the role of a doula and looked into it a bit more.

I contacted Lisa and was very lucky that she happened to be available at late notice to act as our doula. She came and met us and was such a calming and positive presence that we both knew straight away that she was the right person to support us with the birth. Lisa came and met us a couple of times before the birth to get to know us, help us think about and prepare for the birth and talk us through the "What if" scenarios to understand that, although things may happen during the birth outside of our control, what our key aims for the birth were whatever happened, e.g. skin-to-skin immediately after the birth, etc. By talking with her we both felt a lot more prepared.

I also felt comforted that she understood what we were aiming for and could be our spokesperson with anyone else attending the birth, so that I could concentrate on the birth itself. Knowing that Lisa had partnered many women and couples through their births made me feel reassured that an experienced person who knew us and was looking out for our needs would be present when the time came.

I started having contractions late on Monday evening. I was in bed and for each contraction I would go on all fours and breathe through using the Golden Thread Breath, holding the headboard where needed.

By the morning Matt called the homebirth team to give them the heads up and we called our doula Lisa to come over. I started using a TENS machine late morning to help with the contractions. My body was so focused on labour that I was unable to keep anything but water down. Sniffing peppermint oil helped with the nausea.

When the contractions became stronger, I found it helpful to focus on the affirmation "I trust my body to birth my baby" whilst breathing through it. By this time, I was on my knees, rocking back and forward over a gym ball in the lounge.

When the contractions became really strong, so the TENS was no longer so effective, I got in the birth pool in our kitchen/ diner. Matt had done a great job using stick up blackout blinds, electric candles and lots of towels to make it a soothing space. Matt and Lisa massaged my lower back during contractions as I leant on the edge of the pool and changed positions. When I went into labour Lisa was a constant calming, compassionate and reassuring presence and she gave wonderful advice, aromatherapy and fantastic pain-relieving massage too! I would not hesitate to use Lisa again if we were lucky enough to have another baby.

The midwives arrived early afternoon and let me stay in my zone, just keeping a regular check on baby's heartbeat and my pulse. When contractions got stronger still, I asked to use the gas and air and continued to breathe using soft lips and the yoga techniques Tessa taught me.

Things slowed down a little, so I came off the gas and air and just dipped in when I felt I needed it. I started using more vocalisation in yogic breathing and started roaring him out! It took a while for his head to come out, but I could feel it, which gave me the strength to keep pushing. Throughout, his heartbeat was calm and regular. Once his head was out the rest of him followed and I grabbed him and pulled him onto my chest, completely overwhelmed by the achievement and emotion!

We had lovely calm skin-to-skin in the pool and when the cord had gone white, Matt cut it and got his skin-to-skin time too. The placenta took some time to come out, so I got out the pool and managed to deliver it whilst bearing down on the toilet.

We then retreated to a cosy nest on the sofa in our living room for Rory's first breastfeed and more time as a family. It felt like a marathon, but the techniques Tessa taught me during classes and the birth preparation workshop were completely invaluable and helped me achieve the homebirth I wanted.

During Anna's pregnancy, she researched all the options and decided that for her personally, a homebirth would feel like the most soothing place to birth her baby. With the support of her partner and doula, and techniques like the Golden Thread Breath (Box 1), she was able to birth her baby at home. At home, you are in your familiar surroundings and you are more in control of what happens. Midwives step into your territory as they cross the threshold and that shifts the locus of power, for example, with them asking permission to move furniture around. Of course, homebirths are not right for everyone. For some women, particularly where there is a known medical condition, a feeling of safety may only be achieved at the hospital where you know there is the clinical back up.

BOX 1: Golden Thread Breath

Often in birth stories, if a technique is mentioned, it will be the Golden Thread Breath. I learnt this from Uma Dinsmore-Tuli's *Mother's Breath* book.

Settle and observe your breath as it is right now. Start to breathe in through the nose, but out through the mouth. Consciously relax your face, your jaw, your tongue and your lips as you exhale. As you breathe out, imagine a golden thread stretching out across the room in front of you: a very fine, long thread. Feel your body respond with a feeling of relaxation.

The reason we focus on breathing out through the mouth is because there is an intrinsic connection between your jaw/throat area and the pelvic area. As a foetus the cells for these two areas originated in the same place. These two areas act in similar ways and one affects the other. To feel this for yourself, put your thumb in your mouth and be aware of your pelvic floor. Then suck your thumb and feel what happens to the pelvic floor. For most women, there will be a lifting and squeezing feeling.

Ina May Gaskin, an American midwife, calls this 'Sphincter Law'. If you relax the sphincter of the mouth, the sphincter of the cervix will also relax, and dilation will happen more easily. Also, there are three diaphragms in the body: one in the mouth, the respiratory diaphragm, and the pelvic diaphragm. By relaxing the jaw and taking deeper breaths, the first two diaphragms will help the third one to release also.

Whatever you do, keep breathing! Your uterus is a big muscle that needs oxygen to work comfortably and your baby needs oxygen to stay calm. The breath will respond to your body's needs so as contractions intensify, your breathing will become stronger. Practise breathing in more strongly, breathing out a golden rope, perhaps hearing breath now. Later, the breath may be even stronger still and I use the analogy of the huge metal chain that secures a ship to the harbour wall. Remember Anna roaring her baby out!

In between contractions, in the expansion phase, return to the resting Golden Thread Breath. The breathing becoming slow to conserve energy.

Next both a mum and dad tell the story of their son's birth.

SARAH'S BIRTHING STORY

(hypnobirth, episiotomy)

Sarah came throughout her pregnancy to yoga classes and joined the birth preparation workshop with her husband in the third trimester. They had a practical, focused, no-nonsense approach to preparing for the birth with lots of humour evident in their relationship.

Thomas's birth:

On Sunday afternoon a couple of weeks before Easter, we made the finishing touches to the room for our baby and then sat down to watch some TV for the evening. My waters broke in a gush while we were watching "Victoria" on TV, so I was excited and happy that things were happening a week earlier than the due date.

There were no contractions to start with, so we took our time and went into the Rushey [midwife-led] centre for an assessment later that evening. We were told that hopefully I would go into labour in the next 24 hours, otherwise they recommended that they get things started artificially.

We went home and in the early morning the contractions started. I was sick a few times with the stronger contractions. Once they were regular and coming three times in ten minutes, we went into the Rushey centre around 11am, and found out my cervix was 3cm dilated. I was given an anti-sickness injection, and found a quiet area with bean bags to relax in.

About half an hour after arriving there, I felt that the contractions had changed and that I wanted to push. I asked to my husband to "Call the midwife!" and, on reassessment, my cervix was then 10cm dilated so things were happening quickly!

They needed to monitor the baby and we were whisked off to the delivery room and fortunately the signs were good. As he was awkwardly positioned, I had an episiotomy and after that it didn't take long for our baby to be born as he was in a hurry to meet us! Our baby was born at 2.26pm.

He was placed straight onto my tummy and we then found out we had a boy. About five minutes later his cord was cut.

All through the labour I found it incredibly helpful to use the Golden Thread Breath, turning into golden rope and then a heavy golden chain. This kept me focused and calm. In the end there was no time for analgesia. I was glad I had the fantastic support of my husband all through the labour too!

The feeling afterwards was total euphoria.

We stayed in the RBH for a few days to get the hang of breast-feeding and then enjoyed being at home with Thomas feeding well.

Thomas's dad shares his perspective:

I must admit I went to the birth preparation workshop as a slightly doubting husband, sceptical of the real benefits of the hypnobirthing component (was this something like hypnotism that I didn't really like the sound of?), but obviously keen to support my wife!

As the course went on, I began to certainly appreciate that hypnobirthing could help my wife relax and hopefully enable her to find a peaceful state that would help make her experience of childbirth to be a positive one. However, as a soon-to-be first-time father, even then with my naivety, I perhaps couldn't really link these techniques to childbirth or really appreciate how they would help us as a family when it came to the time of the birth. I would find out soon enough.

A few weeks later when my wife went into labour, after our arrival at hospital, it soon became apparent that this wasn't going to be an easy labour with emergency buttons pressed and a team of doctors in the delivery room. At that moment I appreciated that any techniques that were going to help my wife relax for the remainder of the birth would be invaluable – I would take any help we could get!

Accordingly, in the midst of the all the people in the room, the scary arrival of an incubator and serious conversations between the (amazing) medical team, any previous doubts I had about hypnobirthing completely disappeared as my wife used all the breathing techniques to stay incredibly relaxed, focused and able to follow all instructions with amazing clarity and without any panic! She didn't involve herself in the rest of the room's busyness and just focused on her breathing. What a star – I'm so proud of her! With my wife's peaceful approach and the incredible care that we received, our healthy baby son was born.

On reflection, my wife's relaxed, peaceful, focused approach, utilising many of the things she had learned on the birth preparation workshop, can only have helped our baby stay as relaxed as possible in the midst of an otherwise rather dramatic birth! The wonderful medical staff all said the same and were amazed that my wife stayed so calm! It's fair to say that in our moment of need (and now afterwards) I was no longer the doubtful husband, but instead fully appreciative.

Thomas's birth shows how when plans change, it's still possible to have a positive birthing experience. Remaining calm helps the health professionals do their work efficiently and quickly, and the baby is less likely to become distressed by the intervention itself. For some partners, watching a birth – particularly one that has an element of urgency about it – can be the most dramatic experience of their life. They often have better recall of the details of a labour than the mother, who is in a special, even altered state of being due to the hormones circulating.

What I notice in my pregnancy yoga classes is that when we come to the relaxation part at the end, there is occasionally a woman who finds it very difficult to switch off; not closing her eyes, or closing and then flicking her eyes open at the slightest sound, and fidgeting, changing position, or perhaps sighing a lot. Usually as she continues to attend the classes, this will start to change. Her inability to settle is a sign that she is on high alert for some reason. Also, what I observe in classes is that there are some women who feel uncomfortable with closing their eyes when we are practicing breathing techniques or pelvic floor exercises. This is understandable when you are new to a class and everything may feel strange, but when it continues, I wonder whether there is a basic feeling of safety that has been compromised in her life experience. If this resonates in any way with you, gently work with the reflections at the end of this chapter to see how you can transform this.

I always give the option to keep the eyes open, but perhaps to let the eyelids become a little heavier and soften the focus. This is because about 80% of stimulation to the brain is thought to be visual and so this sensory input can be a distraction for many of us when we try to focus on a relaxation technique. By simply closing the eyes, we reduce stimulation to the brain and can make it that much

29

easier to relax. However, if having the eyes open makes someone feel safer, they can do that for as long as is needed. Sometimes a blanket for the relaxation or a change of position in the room can give enough of a feeling of protection to make a difference. The same can be true during the birthing: leaning against the way with your arms around your head or putting a shawl over your head can create a private space even in a busy waiting room.

About five years ago, one of my students arrived at the hospital only for the contractions to fade away. The midwife sent her home until the labour started again. She shared that she just didn't feel ready and was unsettled by the hospital environment. The night after attending one of my birth preparation workshops, she went into labour and her daughter was born the following day. Using techniques like visualising a safe space (Box 2) to keep her nervous system soothed and knowing she could make small, but impactful changes to the hospital room were enough to keep the birthing journey unfolding smoothly this time.

BOX 2: Safe place visualisation

When you think of a place, on some level the brain does not distinguish whether that place is real, a memory or imagined. If it is a place that you associate with calm, relaxation and feeling safe, the body will respond whether you're physically there or not. Read the following text through or record yourself reading it slowly on the voice memo function of your phone.

Make yourself comfortable and close your eyes. Imagine or remember a place where you feel really safe and relaxed. It could be a holiday memory, your favourite place at home or a completely imaginary place. Use all of your senses.

Look around: What do you see in that place? The colours, shapes...

What can you feel? The sun or a breeze on your face, a cosy blanket, your clothing against you...

What sounds can you hear? Or is it quiet?

What can you smell? Outside smells of the sea, or flowers? Inside scents from incense or oils?

What can you taste? What would you have eaten or drunk before you laid down to relax?

Would you like to rest there alone or invite someone to be with you for quiet support?

Notice how you feel.

Every time you're falling asleep from now on, practice coming back to this happy, safe place.

Sometimes women are conscious of what is making them nervous or anxious about the upcoming birth. They may have clear ideas about what will calm them. The concept of 'brakes' and 'accelerators' is useful here for reflecting on what is likely to switch on the sympathetic nervous system (putting brakes on the labour) or the parasympathetic nervous system (moving the birth forwards). The concept originally came from Emily Nagoski's book *Come as You Are*, which is about better understanding the motivators and barriers to sex. Many of the brakes and accelerators are common across sex and birth. If having strangers in the room would put a stop to you feeling comfortable or safe enough to have sex, it's likely it will have the same effect during birth!

Instead, imagine your partner has done the washing up, the lighting is low, you're feeling comfortably warm and unobserved, there's music playing in the background, your partner is using lovely words to encourage you, and you've got all the time in the world. All of these would count as sex accelerators and would aid the birthing journey too. Some women will have very strong brakes and gentle accelerators, others will have weak brakes and powerful accelerators, and every other permutation is possible too. We are all different through our life experiences and personality traits. What may work in one pregnancy, may not in the subsequent one, because our life experiences will have changed in the meantime; we will have changed ourselves.

Shmaila was a student of mine who was pregnant with her third child. She would come to class in a headscarf and remove it once the door was closed and any male partners had left. Towards the end of her pregnancy, she confided in me that she had felt out of control during the labours of her first two children. That night as I was falling asleep, I wondered whether it was an issue of modesty. She had described male doctors coming into the room unannounced and I thought how distressing I would find that when modesty was a core feature of my belief system. When I saw her next, I suggested speaking to the consultant midwife and writing into the birth plan that the health professionals involved in her care would make extra effort to ensure her modesty was maintained. You would hope this would be the case for any woman, but we identified that this would have a particularly deep psychological effect on her and be a massive brake on the labour. This may have contributed to two long previous labours. I also discussed with her partner about how he could act as a modesty barrier if necessary, physically placing himself between her and the door. I'm pleased to share that she felt in control, less exposed and stayed calm the third time around.

We may not always be able to control everything about our environment, but when we address the issues we do have control over, we can shift our frame of mind, stay calm(er) and more empowered.

📖 REFLECTIONS ⟩ on Soothing

Remember dear reader that you do not need to answer all of the questions. You might choose one that feels like a gentle way in or, conversely, the one that you have the biggest reaction to when reading. Choosing what feels like the right way to use these reflections for your inner journey supports you to trust your intuition in other situations.

Would you say, in general, that you go through your days feeling mostly nervous or calm? What sorts of things help to calm you?

What are your 'birthing brakes' and 'birthing accelerators'? (NB. A birthing brake increases stress whereas a birthing accelerator helps you feel calm.) Make a list for both and revisit them as you continue through the pregnancy.

What would really panic you? What steps can you take to deal with those brakes? (e.g. Talking to your midwife about your anxieties, practical solutions like a practice run to the hospital.)

What or whom do you imagine will calm you during labour? What steps can you take to enhance those accelerators? (A second hospital bag filled with things to make a calm space: fairy lights, LED candles, music/relaxation tracks, relaxing oils.)

💡 SUGGESTIONS

Regularly listen to relaxation and/or hypnobirthing tracks, particularly ones created for pregnancy and birth. See www.pearlsofbirthwisdom.com/downloads for a complementary Yoga Nidra.

Use the mindfulness app on your phone.

Soothing movement, including pregnancy yoga, pregnancy pilates, swimming, or a walk in nature.

(Q) **RESOURCES**

Sophie Fletcher (2014) *Mindful Hypnobirthing*. Vermillion, St Ives.

Emily Nagoski (2015) *Come as You Are*. Scribe

https://integratedlistening.com/ssp-safe-sound-protocol/ (If you have particular issues with regulating stress levels, see the Safe & Sound Protocol, which is based on Stephen Porges' excellent research.)

Pearl 2
Feeling Protected

*Simply, we are wired for
Safe or Not Safe.
Every physical or mental
reaction stems from this.*

Imagine you are in a room with the lighting turned down. You were feeling hot, so you only have a baggy T-shirt on, but it's so big that it hangs down and covers your bump and bottom. Your birth partner is between you and the door, creating a buffer between you and the outside world. When the midwife enters the room, you have a moment to adjust to someone else being in your birth bubble. You're leaning forwards, rocking and swaying. You have headphones on and are listening only to what you want to hear. This is the kind of environment that helps a woman feel protected and secure during childbirth.

Now think about the environment many of us have grown up in and the ways that we, as women, have changed the way we behave in order to feel safe. As girls we may have received the message that to be safe, we shouldn't walk home alone in the dark. As women we may wear certain clothes to avoid a certain kind of male gaze. Personally, I find it very hard to fall asleep on trains because somewhere along the line I subconsciously decided I may be too vulnerable. Our past experiences combined with our attitudes about the world play a huge role in our *feelings* of safety. Exploring these feelings is an important part of the birthing journey, as creating a cocoon of safety for birth requires us to feel safe in the world and in our bodies.

Throughout our lives, we are storing memories and creating beliefs about what birth is like. The limbic part of the brain is, simplistically put, a bit like a filing cabinet. Whether we are conscious or not about the effect of our relative's traumatic birth story, the colleagues' admonishment to take all the pain relief going, or the drama of television programme *One Born Every Minute*, our body will react to these stored experiences as a birthing brake. If we witnessed our sibling's straightforward birth at home, the natural birth of our cat's kittens, or read a string of positive birth stories, our body will react to these stored positive experiences as a birthing accelerator.

If the overall balance of your experiences creates a reaction of fear, even subconsciously, the result will be tension in the body and this in turn creates more pain during contractions (Box 3). If instead, there is a feeling that birth can be a natural process and the mother can remain calm and relaxed, she will be able to manage the contractions more comfortably. As a simple example of the physicality of this, hold your hand in front of you and bring tension into the fingers, making a claw shape. Now try to move your hand up and down from the wrist, while maintaining the tension. It gets tiring and uncomfortable very quickly. Now relax your hand, letting it flop down. Again, move your hand up and down from the wrist, while keeping the fingers relaxed. It's so easy and comfortable. Often we talk about the intensity of the surges – they are powerful – they need to be powerful to push your baby out into the world, and so we can reframe them positively.

In our culture currently, the dominant story around birth is that it is painful and dangerous. When we do not question this, our subconscious will react to contractions as a signal that pain and danger are imminent. Hypnobirthing aims to shift the balance, so that our mind allows our body to keep the parasympathetic nervous system (the "rest, digest and birth" system) switched on. This is why it is so important to practice the hypnobirthing tracks through the pregnancy: years of accumulated beliefs may take a while to transform! However, a multipronged approach will be even more powerful. By reading statistics around the safety of different birth locations, for example, we can make an informed decision about the reality of giving birth in different places (e.g.

home, midwife-led centre or delivery suite). By enquiring into our beliefs about birth, we can unpick what is true and what is false, and decide for ourselves where we will feel most protected and safe.

BOX 3: The power of language

In some hypnobirthing courses, the word 'contractions' is replaced with something like 'surges'. I think that this is understandable given the bad press that contractions get. However, as I love anatomy, I have always felt comfortable with the word because that is what the muscles of the uterus (or womb) are doing: contracting. Sometimes when we understand how something works, we can change our reaction to the name.

The uterus has evolved to be this incredible muscular organ that is normally the size of a pear. It grows tremendously during pregnancy to accommodate your baby and shrinks back to its pre-pregnancy size in six to eight weeks after birth. How amazing is that! Just imagine if any part of a man did that, they'd be letting everyone know.

The uterus organ consists of long, round and spiral muscles. During the first stage of labour, the long muscles are contracting to open the cervix (a bit like when you pull a roll neck jumper over your head so that you can see your crown showing through the hole). During the second stage of labour, the round muscles are pushing your baby down and out (similar to the action of squeezing toothpaste out of a tube) and the spiral muscles are turning your baby to pass through the pelvis.

We want the contractions strong and effective so that you can meet your baby sooner. Without artificial hormones, your body is controlling the strength of the hormones and would not make the contractions stronger than you can manage. After each contraction is what I call an expansion phase so that the muscles and you can rest.

Contractions are a testament to just how amazing your body is. Of course, if that word in any way triggers you, please feel free to replace 'contraction' with 'surge' or 'wave' in your mind.

Following are the birthing stories of a two sons three years apart.

EMMA'S BIRTHING STORIES

(quick labours, hypnobirth)

Emma is a petite brunette with intelligent eyes who read voraciously and knew what she wanted.

Oscar's birth:

It was a hot June in 2015 when I was expecting a July baby boy. Aside from the heartburn, the pregnancy had been smooth sailing up until 33 weeks when I developed the signs of pre-eclampsia. Due to high blood pressure, I had to go into hospital a couple of times a week to monitor my baby's heartbeat and the doctors advised that I be induced at 37 weeks. I wanted to avoid an induction, so I tried various attempts to get him moving including bouncing on my birthing ball, eating pineapple and hot things, but I was not having any cramps or aches.

At 36 weeks and 6 days (the day before my induction) I was in hospital for my usual pre-eclampsia checks and the midwife noticed that the baby's heart monitor was showing contractions. I hadn't felt anything other than slight discomfort, so I didn't think anything of it, but they offered to do a sweep considering I was going to have an induction the next day.

During the sweep, the midwife checked my cervix and was sur-

prised I was 4cm dilated and in early labour. She explained that with my condition of high blood pressure it was possible labour was starting naturally faster than normal – even so they sent me home, seemingly confident I would be fine for some time.

Just two hours later, after eating some pizza and watching TV alone whilst my husband did some work in the office upstairs, I started to get stronger pains. I lit some candles around the lounge and leant over my birthing ball whilst watching some documentary about African tribes on the television as the surges started to get closer together. I started timing the contractions but at first they were all over the place, so I gave up thinking it would be many hours before anything really would happen.

I breathed through each contraction, which I had learnt at my yoga class, and just tried to watch the television to keep my mind off things. Then about an hour later the surges were getting stronger and tighter at around six minutes apart, so I asked my husband to come downstairs and then called the hospital, which told me to call back in around an hour if they got down to four minutes.

My instinct was telling me I should be in hospital, but I just put the phone down and went back to pacing around, and about 20 minutes later I was feeling like I needed gas and air. With each wave of contraction, I could not stay still and kept walking around everywhere leaning over the sofa, the dining table and the birthing ball. My husband who was timing the contractions suddenly noticed I was going down to two minutes apart.

He called the hospital, telling them we were going in, and rushed around grabbing our things. At the time I was going to the toilet a lot and noticing a lot of blood, which being my first birth I thought was normal – it is not and was a serious sign of complications. After I was sick in the kitchen sink, I remembered from reading my pregnancy book that this could be the transition stage – a sign I was about to give birth.

As we left the house in a hurry, I had to stop to lean over the car bonnet in pain, trying to just get into the car. By the time we pulled out of our drive I felt the need to push. I remembered in my pre-natal yoga classes being told to pant if I needed to push but shouldn't, so I did that all the way – for 30 minutes to the hospital. We briefly stopped on an A-road layby with trucks for a minute to grab a bottle of water from the boot as I said I felt sick. I did think about getting out of the car and just pushing. It was the most uncomfortable moment in my life to say the least!

When we arrived at the hospital, I was so out of it by this point, almost like I was drunk, I was on another planet and all I could focus on was trying not to push. I imagined I was in my safe place I had been taught at yoga, which for me was a veranda looking out to sea. I managed to tell my husband he needed to get a wheelchair as I could not walk and then I had to be dragged out of the car to the wheelchair and my husband calmly took me up to the delivery suite.

I wasn't screaming in pain, I'm not really one to verbally announce pain and I was so busy focusing on my safe imaginary place to contain the pain that the nurses didn't seem to be concerned when my husband wheeled me in there. Then they took a look at me and everything changed, I remember being told, "Your baby is coming now", and then being wheeled very fast to the delivery room. I leant on the bed on all fours and was told to push straight away, but I didn't know what to do and was feeling tired so they asked me to turn around onto my back. I must not have been listening as I just turned around still on all fours! I eventually managed to get onto my back, and they held a monitor to my bump to keep an eye on him.

I was given gas and air, but I gave up bothering to try it. I tried to push but I wasn't doing it right and then they told me the baby was in distress. All of a sudden it seemed about ten people were in the room and I panicked a little. All breathing techniques went out of window at this point, and they said they would give me a cut to help him come out quicker and then forceps.

I wouldn't listen to the midwife telling me how to push, and I turned to my husband and said I couldn't do it, so he talked me through it and explained if I didn't push now they were getting the forceps. Suddenly I was back in the room and I felt the urge to bear down properly – it was an amazing feeling to push with your body, not against it. He came straight out, surprising the midwife, as I managed to push him out before she could get the doctor with forceps. He was 5lb 1oz.

I felt so proud of my body for delivering him safely and quickly when it was time for him to arrive.

Rupert's birth:

Fast forward three years later and I was expecting another baby boy. Due to my history of pre-eclampsia I was nervous of both complications and another fast birth. I made sure I stayed healthy in pregnancy and kept my blood pressure low and stayed calm, I joined a pre-natal pregnancy yoga class which also had some meditation and hypnobirthing techniques to help with labour.

Because of the complications I had and knowing I struggled at the pushing stage, I was intrigued about how the body naturally does what it needs to do, so I read up on hypnobirthing and bought a hypnobirthing book which came with two CDs – one *had relaxing music for pregnancy and the other music for each labour stage. After many late stage scans, I was released from consultant care as I had no signs of pre-eclampsia and the baby looked to be perfectly healthy – which was a relief.*

I started to consider a hypnobirthing labour with a pool. I did wonder if I should have a homebirth but decided on the hospital just in-case I developed pre-eclampsia at a late stage. I got to 40 weeks and the baby was showing no signs of arriving, I had listened to my hypnobirthing CDs many times over, bounced on the ball a lot and walked around the village and the local woods. I was also on my yoga mat doing some yoga every day to remain calm and read some pregnancy affirmation cards that I put up around the house reminding me I could do this, whatever happens.

As I got close to 41 weeks, I started to feel a lot of pressure on my pelvis including mild aches and cramps that came and went but no sign of labour pains. I tried to eat all the foods to bring on labour and even got my favourite dance music on and jumped around the living room (or wobbled with a 41-week bump). Every night before I went to bed, I would listen to my hypnobirthing CD and it would send me off to a calm relaxing sleep – well before I would have to get up to the toilet in the middle of the night.

At my 41-week midwife appointment she checked me and said I was already 4cm and did not know how I was not already in labour! I remembered from my previous pregnancy that usually my body waits till the last minute before all systems go. I had a sweep and had a relaxing evening at home. The following day in the afternoon I went to the bathroom and noticed my plug had given away – something which never happened with my first pregnancy. I felt like my body was telling me it was going to happen very soon – although at this point I had no other signs of labour.

I went to bed listening to my mediation CD at 9pm and was woken up at 12.30am with what felt like I might have constipation and so I went to the toilet sat down and a huge wave of contraction started. I came straight out and woke my husband up saying I was in labour and asked him to get the birthing ball.

As I leant over the birthing ball on my knees in our bedroom the contractions came thick and fast, we timed them, and they were already 2 minutes apart. My husband called his parents to come babysit our 3-year-old (they were on call to come at a minute's notice). He also called the delivery suite but apparently couldn't get through, I thought about shouting at him to make sure he got the number right but the waves of contractions were intense and I was trying to concentrate on my breathing – Breathing in whilst saying in my head 'I am calm' and Breathing out 'I am calm, I am relaxed'.

As his parents walked in the door, I felt a huge pop and a massive gush of water came down my legs as my waters had broken. Just after I changed into my birthing gown, I felt sick and managed to get my husband to grab a bowl before I threw up. I remembered this was it – the transition phase and it was only about 45 minutes after my contractions started! I had previously had discussions with my husband about the possibility of a fast labour and I said if I am sick and if I feel the need to go the hospital we have to go. So I told him we needed to go and straight out the door we headed.

He eased me into the front seat, put on some gentle music and I tried to maintain my calm breathing (I am calm, I am calm and relaxed) during each contraction whilst focusing on the hypnobirthing technique of noticing the senses (the feel of the car, the lights of the road, the cold fresh air). I tried to just zone out as much as I could, luckily it was only a 10-minute drive to the hospital.

When we arrived at the hospital my husband got a wheelchair

45

for me and we went straight to delivery, the midwife was calm and said it was the night everyone seemed to be having babies and put us in a waiting room whilst she went to see to someone else. The contractions were intense at this point and I was squeezing my husband's hand ever so tightly. He reminded me to keep breathing and focusing, I was finding it hard with the bright lights and all my instincts were telling me to go on all fours and they wanted me on my back to check my cervix to see how far I was dilated.

After what felt like forever but probably wasn't, they checked my cervix and told me I was 10cm and ready to push – I felt like screaming at them I knew this already. They whizzed me off in the bed to the delivery room where it was dark and calm, and I immediately relaxed and went straight onto all fours leaning over the massive pillows.

I took in a deep breath of gas and air and I have to say it was such a relief after dealing with the intense contractions. I immediately drifted off to my safe place – imagining I was on a beach with the waves lapping at my feet. I could hear the midwife talking to me and I listened as she told me to "Just let your body do what it feels it needs to do" and so I relaxed and let my body push him out as I breathed deeply. With each contraction I took in a breath of gas and air and as I breathed out I let my body push him out a bit more.

I heard the midwife and my husband say they could see the head and I gave one final push. It was just 10 whole minutes of pushing and he was fully out and crying in between my legs. My 7lb 11oz healthy baby boy went straight to the breast and we laid there for ages in total calm with each other. Labour lasted just 2 hours and 30 minutes and it was the calmest loveliest birth I could have hoped for.

In both of Emma's births, she managed her fast labours incredibly with techniques that calmed her, including going to her safe place (Box 2, previous chapter) and using the resting breath (Box 4). The relaxation and breathing techniques may not remove the pain entirely, but they can make the intensity of the contractions or surges more manageable and increase the amount of time before you need pain relief. They can also enable you and your birth partner to stay calm if something unexpected happens or labour is happening faster than you thought or when intervention is required. This enables the health professionals to focus on supporting you more quickly.

BOX 4: Resting breath

Settle into a comfortable position and notice your breath. As you breathe in, slowly count 1, 2, 3. As you breathe out, slowly count 1, 2, 3, 4. Gradually lengthen the breath so that you may count to 5 or 6 on the exhalation, if that feels comfortable. The focus is on lengthening the exhalation in relation to the inhalation to signal to the nervous system that you are safe and relaxed. The number you reach does not matter so keep the breathing easy.

Some people prefer counting as it keeps their mind gently occupied. Others prefer words. Try breathing in, saying mentally "Breathing in I am calm", and as you breathe out, say mentally "Breathing out, I am calm, I am relaxed". Keep this going as long as you want to.

In the next story, Teresa describes the births of her two children.

TERESA'S BIRTHING STORIES

(active birth, gas and air)

Teresa is a dynamic woman, with a zest for life and new experiences. I think like me, if she believes that something will be good for her, she will put 110% effort into the experience.

Alex's birth:

At the beginning I wasn't sure how the yoga lessons were helping me. Tessa was always talking about positions during the labour, to find a visual happy place, and to have a focus sentence [affirmation] that you could use during that moment. I was only 18 weeks, so I doubted that it could benefit me. But I kept going to every Saturday lesson, because I truly believe in yoga. Something I didn't consider and realised after a few lessons was how lucky I was to have found an amazing community.

Every Saturday I used to walk 20 minutes to Caversham. I started to understand what Tessa was telling us, putting it in practice. Also, I started to be part of the "Mummies community", enjoying my time with other mums who were having similar experiences, joys and pains.

The night that the contractions started I was 39 weeks. I woke up at 1.30am. I was feeling a little different to normal. I ob-

served a little bit of 'water' after I went to the toilet. At 3.30am I decided to call the midwife's number at the hospital, because I continued to observe more and more water. They advised me to take a shower and to go to the hospital in a few hours. One hour later, I asked my husband to leave to the hospital because I was having contractions more often.

The most useful exercise was leaning forwards against the wall (legs straight, hands on the wall and moving from one side to the other one. Because my bump was 'hanging' forwards, the contractions were better). The breathing technique I used the most (at the same time as the posture) was to breath in and out thinking of the sentence Tessa advised us to keep in mind: "Breathing in I am calm, breathing out I am calm, I am relaxed". I had my son at around 7.30am.

I know, I was one of those "lucky" ladies who had a great birth. But I can't take all the credit. Tessa was in my mind most of the time. Thanks to her advice, the affirmations and the exercises, I could go through the pain in an easier way. I also felt that my body was ready and that it knew what to do.

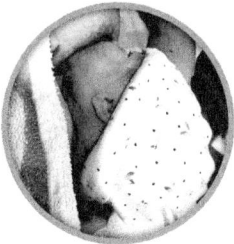

Sofia's birth:

My waters started breaking on Thursday night. It wasn't massive, just a little bit of water. I went to sleep, because I wasn't having contractions. I woke up Friday at 4am and I found more water (still a little bit). Also, I was having contractions without pain.

I remembered Tessa's advice, so I decided to rest and dis-

tract myself by watching a good movie. At 7am I decided to drop off my son to nursery and go to work, because the contractions stopped. Because I saw more water (again it wasn't much), on our way to work I called the triage. They asked me about my contractions and about the water. Because of my previous quick delivery, they decided to check the water and the baby's condition, so they asked me to go to the hospital.

At around 11am they decided to send me home for no more than 24 hours, because I dilated 3cm and I wasn't having frequent contractions ... I decided to distract myself and to rest, because I'd need the energy.

One hour later the contractions started again. It was easy to decide to go to the hospital, because I followed your advice that active labour is started when "I needed to stop and concentrate on my breathing in each contraction". This one was one of the best advices I've learned with you!

When I arrived, I was already 5cm dilated so they asked me to stay. Because my water wasn't broken the process was a little slow. I stood up, kept breathing with my hands on the bed and allowing the tummy to hang, helping with the pain. Also, I repeated my sentence "Keep calm, trust your body. It knows what to do." That position and the mantra helped me to concentrate on the breathing.

After an hour, the contractions were more painful, so I asked my midwife to measure how far was I, because I was considering requesting the epidural. They offered me the gas and air to help me go through the contractions and to give them the time to call for the epidural. While they were measuring me, the waters broke fully. I was 6cm so I decided to ask for the epidural. I knew that I would need my energy for later.

Luckily, everything escalated and the second stage started quickly. I didn't have time for the epidural but using gas and air only I had Sofia 30 minutes later.

Teresa started at home, like most mothers do, and then moved to the midwife-led unit at the local hospital. The posture she describes in the first birthing (upright , leaning forwards against the way) is one that we practice weekly in class, because it is so effective in taking the edge off the intensity of the surges. This is particularly true if you are experiencing them mainly in your back. (Sometimes there is an assumption that you will feel the contractions at the front of your body because that's where the bump is, but, remember, the uterus has round and long muscles that surround your baby. Depending on how the baby is positioned you may actually feel the intensity more towards the back of your body.) I loved that she rested in the early part of the birthing journey because I know that's against her nature! What I particularly like about Theresa's story is her connection to the community of expectant mothers. As someone living away from her home country, the sense of protection can come from knowing there is a support network around you, and that fuels a can-do attitude.

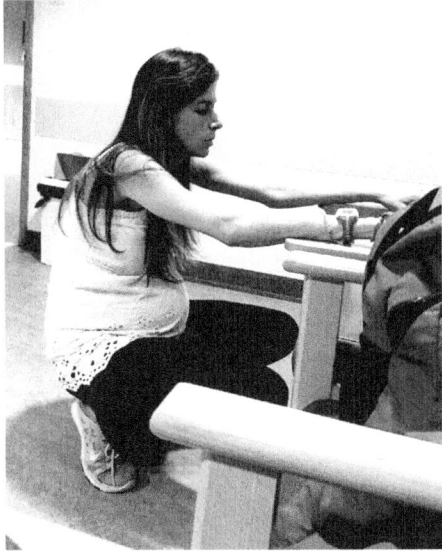

At a women's circle recently, I asked the participants to share the story of their own birth. More than half, despite having their own children, had no idea of what their mothers' birthing stories were, apart from the date they were born. I wondered why this would be.

Is it that we are subconsciously fearful of the story and its effect if it's negative? Do we think that birth care has changed so much that it won't be relevant to our experience?

There is a wonderful story told by Anna Verwaal, a Dutch Maternal-Child Health nurse, whose passion in life is the impact of the birth journey on the baby. In her TED talk she tells how she was once travelling to the airport in a taxi and the driver was obviously uncomfortable with his shirt collar being done up, as he kept pulling at it. She asked about it and he said that he'd always been the same and was dreading his daughter's wedding where he was expected to wear a formal shirt and tie. Anna asked whether he knew about his own birth and perhaps his umbilical cord had been wrapped around his neck. It turns out that it was, three times. Our bodies store a memory of our birth and this can subconsciously impact how we approach the births of our own children for better or for worse. Sometimes simply by acknowledging what has happened to you and knowing that you have different knowledge or support from what your mother had, is enough to release the effect. Sometimes support from an experienced facilitator like Anna Verwaal is useful.

When most women do not have a consistent midwife or a doula, as in most places in the UK, the protection of the birth space tends to fall on the shoulders of the birth partner. With a first baby, many birth partners have never been in that role and are frankly totally unprepared for what that might entail if they have not read birth stories or been on a practice-based course. In the birth preparation workshops I run, there is often an expectation among students that the midwife will guide the couple throughout the journey from first contraction to first feed. While this is realistic for some couples, others find themselves surprised by how little guidance they have during parts of the birth journey, particularly during early labour.

In the birthing of my first daughter, which you will read later in this book, my wonderful midwife did guide us beautifully, but only once we were at hospital. There were hours of labour before that point. If the labouring woman and her birth partner are unprepared for the realities of early labour, this can become a time of anxiety and create more painful contractions. Instead of a slow build of contractions before care of a doctor or midwife become available, it can feel very isolating and create panic if you are not prepared.

A birth partner may need to protect the birthing woman psychologically in addition to physically making a birth space conducive to feeling safe (e.g. low lighting, music or a relaxation track playing in the background, monitor turned away with the volume down). At one point, a student from my classes named Carolina said that a consultant insisted on talking through each contraction, despite her saying in between contractions (in the expansion phase) that the distraction made it much harder to manage the intensity of them and to stop doing that. She said that the consultant was talking about a non-urgent situation and she wished that her husband had protected her birthing space.

Many partners are not expecting to be in this role of protector, or are even aware of the role, or what they are trying to protect. However, they can learn! The Relaxation Deepener technique is wonderful for feeling that someone is totally present for you (see box). This is where a doula or any person who has experience of the importance of the feeling of safety in birth and of protecting the birth 'bubble' is invaluable. Think carefully about resources here: is it worth investing in someone experienced in attending births who can travel with you on the journey, one that you will remember your whole life, or expecting your partner, who may or may not have experience in this area, to be your main support? The answer will vary based on your past experiences with your partner and how they feel about supporting you in this way.

Box 5: Relaxation Deepener

Ask your partner to read through these instructions first. Partner – you will need to be able to see her chest rising and falling in time with her breath.

Say "Sit or lie comfortably with your eyes closed. Take some slow, deep breaths."

(Wait until you can see her breathing out with the chest falling) and say "Nine".

(Chest falls again): "Eight. You are relaxing more and more."

(Chest falls again): "Seven. You are becoming calmer."

(Go at the speed of her breathing. Chest falls again): "Six. Your arms and legs are heavy."

(Chest falls again): "Five. Your breathing is slowing down."

(Chest falls): "Four. You are feeling so much more relaxed."

(Chest falls): "Three. Well done, you are doing so well."

(Chest falls): "Two. Letting go as much as you want to."

(Chest falls): "One. Every muscle and fibre of your body is relaxing."

(Chest falls): "Zero. You are deeply relaxing now."

You can then repeat the whole process as many times as you need to. Feel free to change the affirmations – you can ad lib as you feel more comfortable. Make sure that you slow down the counting as her breath slows down, matching her pace. If you dissolve into giggles the first few times, don't worry. Practice makes perfect. Well done!

REFLECTIONS on Feeling Protected

With all the reflection exercises in this book, I suggest you write as a stream of consciousness in response to the questions. You can read back over what you have written and draw out the main insights.

Have you explored the different locations you could birth your baby? What are they? Where did you think you would feel most comfortable and why? Has that changed after reading more information? (See also resource list)

If you are not birthing at home, how can you change the atmosphere of the place where you are giving birth to create a feeling of protection? What things can you take into hospital to create a more familiar, calm space? (E.g. A sign for the door saying 'Hypnobirth in progress. Quiet please'; headphones so you listen to the sounds that support you.)

Discuss the role of the protector with your birth partner. Do they feel able to fulfil that role? What can help them prepare for that role?

If you can, ask your mother about your own birth. (This can have a tremendous subconscious effect on how your body will respond. I strongly recommend watching Anna Verwaal's TED talk (see below) to understand how your birth affects you into adulthood.)

💡 SUGGESTIONS

If you are preparing for a hospital birth, create a separate hospital bag full of things that can create a calm space. Really go to town on this! If you are preparing for a homebirth, consider how you will protect your calm environment, e.g. turning off from unneeded devices/phones, preventing interruptions from deliveries or un- expected visitors. Reflect on who you are 100% comfortable with being at the birth.

Include information in your birth plan/preferences about how you want the room to be.

Read positive birth stories by yourself and with your partner.

🔍 RESOURCES

www.tellmeagoodbirthstory.com

Leah Hazard (2011) *Father's Homebirth Handbook*. Pinter & Mar- tin. (The homebirth resources are great for positive stories even if you're not planning a homebirth.)

Natalie Meddings (2017) *Why Homebirth Matters*. Pinter & Martin.

Homebirth groups (on Facebook or in person), even if you're not planning on a homebirth you can learn a lot about physiological birth.

Ina May Gaskin (2003) *Ina May's Guide to Childbirth*. Bantam Dou- bleday Dell.

Anna Verwaal's TED talk 'From Womb to World' (www.youtube. com/watch?v=bZ6gLGCy840)

Jennifer Hollowell et al. (2016) 'Women's birth place preferences in the United Kingdom: a systematic review and narrative synthesis of the quantitative literature.' *BMC Pregnancy Childbirth.* 16: 213. (Open access to whole article: https://www.ncbi.nlm.nih.gov/pmc/articles/PMC4977690/)

Vanessa Scarf et al. (2018) 'Maternal and perinatal outcomes by planned place of birth among women with low-risk pregnancies in high-income countries: A systematic review and meta-analysis.' *Midwifery.* 62: 240-55. (Open access to whole article: https://www.sciencedirect.com/science/article/pii/S0266613818300974)

Pearl 3
Embodiment

*Experiences gathered through
our lifetime determine how
comfortable our own bodies feel.*

*Acknowledging the body's
intelligence underpins our ability
to trust the journey of birth.*

Imagine a young child playing. She innocently moves around, belly sticking out as she stands, suddenly running as the impulse takes her, then laying down on the ground when tired. As we get older, the body becomes constrained and self-conscious in a myriad of ways. We have to sit at desks at school, moulding our posture. We override the urge to go to the toilet, waiting for the break. Shoes with thick soles stop sensations being felt in the feet. We draw in our tummies and tuck our tailbones under to show a more svelte silhouette. We ignore our exhaustion and push on.

After reaching adolescence, many women spend the first part of their lives fearful of becoming pregnant (when they are not ready to start a family) or of catching a sexually transmitted disease. Surveys about sex education in secondary schools repeatedly find that it is considered 'too little, too late and too biological'. The pupils want more about the reality of being in relationship with others and the role of pleasure, rather than scaremongering. It is my belief that the fear of pregnancy can become so deep-rooted that even when a woman later wants to conceive a baby, the body blocks this possibility. A yoga nidra (relaxation track) that I created for fertility to reverse this fear and give permission to the body to conceive has been happily successful among my clients.

We become disconnected from the body in other ways too, particularly in relation to our wombs. In women's circles, I have heard countless times how when a girl's period started, she felt let down by her body because she wouldn't be able to keep up with the boys. Despite the wave of period positivity, the taboo around menstruation means that many women put up with debilitating pain in silence. The average time to get a diagnosis for endometriosis is still seven years, because women are not believed about the level of pain they are experiencing. As women, we may have internalised the feeling that our bodies are somehow dysfunctional – what with leaky, crampy periods and the possibility of getting pregnant at the wrong time – and so we come to distrust our own bodies and instead trust doctors, drugs and hospitals to fix us. In this way we may have disconnected from our own bodies and handed over the control to others.

By reconnecting with our bodies and healing from past disconnection, we create a possibility to develop a deep trust of our capabilities. Imagine a dancer who through training can trust the movements available to her, improvise new expressions or dance without consciously thinking of every step. We can relinquish the control of the mind and follow our physical instincts. Or an athlete who prepares mentally, as well as physically for the race: visualising strength, resilience and crossing the finishing line with finesse. We can have confidence in our bodies to achieve great things like birth and normal things like birth.

Following are two different stories of embodiment: a vaginal birth after caesarean (VBAC) and the inner journey taken from a first to second birthing.

SARANYA'S BIRTHING STORY

(VBAC, long first stage)

Saranya is a reserved Indian woman who shared with me that she had found the birth of her first child, a son, difficult because she had felt out of control. It had ended in a caesarean birth and she hoped that this time would be different. She found her second pregnancy hard going because of pelvic pain, but she was determined to practice anything that would help.

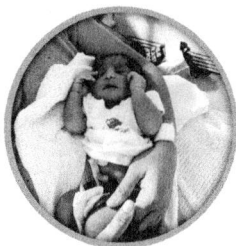

Diya's birth:

I felt strange Braxton hicks on Monday. On Tuesday morning, the contractions started to regularly [come] six minutes apart [and] last for 50 seconds. We called triage but were told to wait for three-minute contractions. I managed the pain with the golden thread breathing. By Wednesday, the contractions became ten minutes apart but lasted for 50 seconds to one minute.

We went to triage for an assessment. I was 2cm dilated. We went home and I had a nice shower and fruit juices. Again, we went to triage around 3pm and I was 5cm dilated.

The midwife in triage quickly checked the baby's position, engagement and heartbeat then sent me to the delivery suite. I always wanted to try the birth pool and I was allowed to use it.

There, I enjoyed the warm water and breathed with the contractions. Within three hours my body took control and wanted to push. The midwife asked me to try different position to help baby to rotate. I don't know where I got all the energy from. After a long few pushes, she was placed on my chest and we had nice skin-to-skin cuddles.

I can't thank you enough for teaching us amazing techniques and spreading the positivity. Last week you told me this time labour going to be different. Indeed, it was different, and I can't be more happy.

My baby girl, Diya, was born on January 29 and shares her birthday with daddy. She weighed 3.1 kg.

Saranya could so easily have lost confidence in her body's ability to birth her baby through a long first stage of labour. However, through yoga she found a way to listen to her body and trust again that birth was a natural process. VBACs can be such a healing journey: a reclamation of something that was missing from her caesarean birth. This is not to say that something is always lost during a caesarean birth, it is the individual journey that determines the experience.

ZIVILE'S BIRTHING STORIES
(active births)

Zivile is a health professional and likes to be prepared. In her first pregnancy, I think she prepared as she would have for her final exams at university: very much an intellectual exercise. For the second birth, she had a different approach...

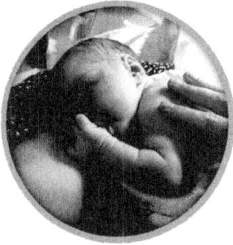

Jasmine's birth:

I would like to share my experience of the birth of my two children. The birthing journey was not just a simple life event. It was my personal growth journey as well.

When I was pregnant the first time, I did not know what to expect from the labour and birth. All my knowledge and imagination were made from stories I heard, books I read, internet I searched, advice I listened to. The only thing I knew [was] that I wanted the birth to happen in as natural a way as possible.

So I started my preparation. I was like a student: I wanted to collect as much information as I could, I wanted to learn all possible techniques that I could choose and use them in the time of birthing. As soon as I was 12 weeks pregnant, I searched for any exercise classes for the pregnant women. Physically I was very inactive [before my pregnancy]. I did believe that by being physically weak you will not be able to deliver your baby.

I found a yoga class which suited me the best with the time and location. "Alright", I thought, "that does not require lots of energy and gives some strength. I am in!". I really liked our teacher, Tessa, since day one. She did everything with a huge passion and she accepted every woman with a pure wisdom.

In the yoga class I enjoyed meditation and, following Tessa's advice, I started doing meditation on a daily basis. I felt ready for birthing as I had so much knowledge (I felt like a student well prepared for her exams). I even made the birth plan with my midwife. At week 41, labour started. We went to hospital despite over-the-phone advice to stay at home a bit longer. As soon as we were there, my waters broke.

The midwife told me, "Your ketone levels are too high, your baby's heart rate is weak, and you will not deliver yourself". I felt really upset as I was SO ready, but I was not ready for this. I was in the theatre, lying in the usual legs-up position, vulnerable and scared. Vaginal examinations were so uncomfortable. All my learning and pre-natal course knowledge was out through the window. I was just breathing. In the theatre, the doctor gave me a few tries to deliver naturally: "You need to be quick – otherwise we are doing c-section". I was more stressed and tense.

My eyes met the eyes of the midwife on my right – probably she saw fear and panic in me. She guided me so well and precisely; she calmed me just by looking at me with understanding eyes. In the end I did deliver naturally. I did not use any medication, nor gas. I did have an episiotomy and lots of stitches. All my body ached so much. I was happy cuddling our healthy baby girl.

After some time, I re-thought my birthing. My friend shared her personal experience when she struggled to deliver, and she was even more prepared than me. I realised that I was not ready at all. I realised that my mind was ready, but my body was not. I realised that I did not give my body any chance to take over and do it from inner wisdom. I did not trust my body to birth.

Bernard's birth:

When I became pregnant the second time, I rushed to Tessa's yoga class. With the second pregnancy I had been gifted with an inner knowledge. This time I knew that I do not need strength to deliver our baby, I do not need knowledge to deliver our baby, I do not need a birth plan to deliver our baby. Birth is something beyond logic. I was listening to birthing stories with different feelings. Before the first birth, hearing women's positive stories about labour and birth did not help me to feel better. I was questioning myself: "She did it, but would I be able to do so well?". Second time I knew that EVERY SINGLE BIRTH is different, and you cannot compare anything.

I was doing yoga poses consciously: I listened to my body's limits and skipped some exercises which did not feel right for my body. First time, I pushed myself to do all the poses as I wanted to be stronger and more flexible. Meditation and breathing were the most valuable tools (and they still are in raising our kids). It gave me inner peace. It shifted me into my inner wisdom. It calmed my mind, it quieted my mind. Meditation and breathing helped me to stay in myself even if situations were not going the way I wanted.

Second time, I did not concentrate about 'outer' things (birthing plans, expectations, baby gender, readings, etc.), but I concen-

trated on how to communicate with my body and my inner wisdom. At week 39 my waters broke, and we went to the hospital. It happened to be the Bank holiday weekend. My midwife did not welcome us. I felt like she just wanted to go home.

I was told: "Your and your baby's heart rate is too fast and we need to perform a c-section". I was in the theatre. The doctor decided to try with IV fluids first. It worked. They postponed the c-section. Then there was a shift change, and we had a new midwife. She was a blessing from Heaven. She believed in my ability to give birth. My body relaxed. She did not do any vaginal examination. She allowed me to lie how I felt the best.

I was in tune with my body and my body gave me signals where to press most. Back pressure points and positions I have known – none worked for me. My body showed different areas to be pressed. With stronger contractions, I felt a need to be pressed stronger into those pressure points. I asked my husband to do it as I could not press any harder.

I did not have much pain at all. I did not use any medication nor gas. I felt baby moving through the birth canal and relaxed my body even more. I was not pushing hard at all, I was just helping my body to do its job. I felt so well and fit after birthing. It was such a different experience. I was happy cuddling our healthy baby boy.

My personal birthing experience was a nice journey towards realisation that YOU CANNOT BE READY FOR EVERYTHING, BUT YOU CAN BE READY TO ACCEPT ANYTHING THAT MIGHT HAPPEN. The most important knowledge lies deep within us. Accepting everything with gratitude gives you relaxation (in your mind and in your body) and makes birthing easier. Second time, I had more stressful and unexpected situations, but I was more relaxed and more in tune with my body. I could easily have fallen into a stress cycle and become tense. I trusted my body and did not disturb it.

I really wish that more and more women have this natural trust in their abilities to give birth and less fear in this magical life event.

I am in awe of Zivile's personal journey. Given what I wrote at the start of this chapter, I sometimes feel it's a big ask of someone to move from what may be decades of mistrust in their body (e.g. from fear of falling pregnancy or painful periods) to trusting in the natural process of birth. However, when they are dedicated to self-reflection this is totally possible and I have seen it time and again.

The inner journey is not often acknowledged in pregnancy classes and so someone may diligently attend antenatal yoga classes, listen to hypnobirthing tracks and take part in the childbirth education, but miss that birth is a rite of passage for a reason. It asks a lot of us, usually in ways we were not expecting. Commonly, it is with a second pregnancy that I find women really engage with the inner process because they comprehend the journey ahead. And there are others that resolutely ignore all of this and that's okay too. In the end, I can guide women in preparing for the journey, but I cannot take that journey for them. There is the potential not only for the birth of a baby, but also the birth of a wiser, more self-aware woman and mother.

As a yoga teacher, I have seen disconnection from the body or specific parts of the body many times. In pregnancy yoga, there is an exercise we do standing against the wall. We bend the knees and slide down the wall slightly. We move the pelvis forwards and backwards, so that the lower back is away from the wall and then gently pushed into it, rocking forwards and backwards. Sometimes the conscious ability to move the pelvis separately from the rest of the body is simply not there, but it can be learned. Also, there is sometimes a total confusion about the pelvic floor and an inability to locate different parts. Again, this can be learnt through intention and practice (see box).

BOX 6: Listening to the body

A simple, but powerful method of reconnecting with the body and fundamentally respecting her, is to become mindful of what your body needs. In class, I always do this as the relaxation is finishing: "Before you move, ask yourself what the body is asking for. Is it to be still a little longer? Is it to have a stretch or move into a new position? Is it to drink more water today or have a nap after lunch?"

Once you've read this, close your eyes and enquire what your body wants to tell you. Deeply listen. Perhaps you've been sitting in one position too long. Perhaps you really need a wee and have been putting off going. Maybe you're ready for a cup of tea.

Listening to the body's cues supports you during labour by indicating what will make you as comfortable as possible. Maybe it just feels better to have your left leg forwards in that standing position you're in (it could be where your baby's head is pushing on a nerve and the change in position will let your baby move). Perhaps you feel like you're on another planet and someone holding your ankles grounds you. Maybe normally you love massage, but touch is distracting you from focusing on the sensations inside your body.

Practice this powerful mindfulness exercise a few times a day so it becomes second nature.

(NB there may also be times when a midwife suggests something that you really don't feel like doing that will help! Like when you're comfortable in the birthing pool and she wants you to get out for a wee, otherwise the full bladder is blocking your baby coming out. This is where trust in your caregiver plays an important role.)

In the pregnancy classes, I talk about the evidence for perineal massage reducing tears in first vaginal births. The perineum is the diamond of tissue going from front to back of the pelvis, and from side to side from the ischial spines (end of the sitting bones), to create the underneath of you. There are often giggles or a look of squeamishness, and sometimes revulsion, about the idea of touching this part of the body. I'm not sure if it's because the perineum is seen as a purely sexual part of the body that is being taken out of context, or touching yourself is not something you talk about, or touching yourself in itself is taboo. What I do wonder is how, if it's so difficult to imagine doing the perineal massage, will the mind-body react if a midwife touches that area to help birth the baby or support the tissue? For example, a compress held to the side of the crowning baby's head has been shown to prevent tearing.

If there has been sexual trauma, please speak to your midwife so health professionals who have expertise in supporting women with this experience can co-create a birth plan that will take this into account. Even if there is not trauma, but discomfort, here is an opportunity to create a healthy connection with this amazing part of our anatomy. In mother and daughter circles that I run around the time of puberty, I suggest giving the girls hand mirrors so that they can look at their vulva. This can be a first step in familiarising yourself with your own genitalia. Then, you might sit for a few days with the intention of touching the perineum (but without actually touching). Sit with the feelings that come up and as a good friend of mine says, feel the feels. If there is emotional discomfort, let it be there. Name it. If there is shame, disgust, fear..., let it be there. Name it. And utilise Brené Brown's books and TED talks to understand more about these feelings (see Resources below). When (if) you feel ready, move on to the perineal massage itself (see box).

BOX 7: Perineal massage

From my perspective, this is as much about becoming comfortable with your vulva as it is about the elasticity of the tissue. Find a lubricant that will not irritate the delicate skin and apply it to a washed thumb or index finger. Get into a position where you can reach between your legs easily: this might be lying down or with one leg lifted on a chair (or side of the bath). Insert the thumb or finger into the vulva (which leads up to the vagina) and push firmly back towards the anus and then make a horseshoe-shaped motion from side to side.

This may feel tingly but should not be painful. Continue for up to a few minutes, building up over time. If difficult feelings arise, stop and feel them. Use the Golden Thread breath if needed, to soothe and calm. (If necessary, seek support for difficult feelings from your midwife or self-refer to Talking Therapies making sure you tell them that you are pregnant.)

Birth is an intimate occasion. Where there has been a natural conception, many of the factors that helped you conceive will support you also in birthing. Low lighting, low voices/music/quiet, comfort, warmth, gentle touch, movement. All these things support the release of oxytocin, variously called the shy, private or love hormone. Imagine trying to poo with lights in your face, strangers standing around your bottom and the door open to a corridor. Not conducive! Birth is no different. Oxytocin and adrenalin work diametrically to one another, like a seesaw: if stress levels increase and adrenalin rises, the oxytocin will decrease and contractions fade. Creating a safe, private and intimate space can be achieved in different places but can be harder in a delivery suite. The birth partner will need to work harder to protect the birth bubble, but it is totally possible when you have thought how you will achieve this and prepared for it.

If you can be comfortable with your body and the body's intelligence is respected, the intricate interplay of hormones necessary for natural birth can unfold smoothly. Where there is shame, mistrust or sensed danger, a locking down will understandably happen. Feeling safe enough to open physically is fundamental. There are simple solutions to help you provide a sense of privacy, such as retreating to the toilet which is a smaller room and cannot contain lots of people, using a birth pool which creates a 'skirt' of privacy below water, or even using a shawl over your head so that people aren't directly watching you and you can avoid a feeling of self-consciousness. This is particularly important as the baby is crowning, as you may be hypersensitive at this time to any comments about progress.

It is comforting to know that the baby can be an active participant in birth, pushing his or her legs to help move through the birth canal. Babies 'know' to be head down ready for birth. There is usually a reason if they are breech or transverse, like tight ligaments within the mother's body affecting the space available to move in the womb. Many of my pregnant clients have had great success with turning breech babies with chiropractors who specialise in the Webster technique, which can create the needed space.

📖 REFLECTIONS ⟩ on Embodiment

Remember you can pick one question to reflect on. Be kind and patient with yourself if you are resistant.

How do you view your body – negatively or positively? Do you trust or mistrust your body? Why?

How do you feel about the changes that pregnancy is bringing to your body?

Who knows more about your body or how to fix/manage it? (you, a partner, a health professional?) Does this change as you read more about how your body works in birth? How?

How does the prospect of showing your genitals to health professionals make you feel? How does a smear test make you feel? Could anything make this easier?

(E.g. for a smear test you can take a chaperone to the appointment, during birth you can decline vaginal examinations that are optional and opt for a water birth if possible so the water creates a buffer. There is research evidence that a vaginal examination (VE) on arrival at hospital will decrease the likelihood of intervention later on, but further VEs do not help in assessing when the baby is likely to be born.)

💡 SUGGESTIONS

Perineal massage (this can also help with previous scarring, e.g. from an episiotomy, but there are also professionals that are trained to work with scar tissue to make it more comfortable and less rigid). Further instructions on perineal massage can be found at www.weleda.co.uk/perineal-massage

Listen to hypnobirthing or yoga nidra tracks that describe how amazing your body is.

RESOURCES

Brené Brown. *I Thought it Was Just Me (But it Isn't)*. (Or see her TED talk on 'The Power of Vulnerability' at www.youtube.com/watch?v=iCvmsMzlF7o)

Blandine Calais-Germaine (2003) *The Female Pelvis*. Eastland Press. (For anatomy lovers like me.)

Uma Dinsmore-Tuli (2014) Yoni Shakti. *YogaWords Ltd*. (Many yoga practices for connecting to the female body and a chapter specifically on pregnancy.)

Uma Dinsmore-Tuli (2006) *Mother's Breath: A Definitive Guide to Yoga Breathing, Sound and Awareness Practices for Pregnancy, Birth, Post-natal Recovery and Mothering*. Sitaram and Sons.

Bessel van der Kolk (2015) *The Body Keeps the Score: Mind, Brain and Body in the Transformation of Trauma*. Penguin. (Excellent book about the cause, effect and treatment of trauma.)

Richard Strozzi-Heckler (2014) *The Art of Somatic Coaching: Embodying Skillful Action, Wisdom, and Compassion*. North Atlantic Books.

Naomi Wolfson (2013) *Vagina: A New Biography*. Virago.

Abby Normal (2018) *Ask Me About My Uterus*. Nation Books. (One woman's journey to reclaim her body with endometriosis.)

Pearl 4
Moving Freely

*As vibrational and physical
beings, we are constantly
moving like everything else
in this universe.*

Traditionally, belly dancing was not a performance art – it was a sacred dance for women to enjoy together in preparation for childbirth. Imagine a belly dancer surrounded by her female friends and family, all moving together like a flock of starlings: synchronised and graceful. Her hips moving hypnotically from side to side. It feels good to move, natural and feminine. Later, when the same woman is birthing her child, she dances unself-consciously through her labour, easing and quickening the birth process.

This image is different from what most of us picture when we think of a labouring woman. Birthing has become very medical-ised, and many of our norms present challenges for both mother and baby. Typically, on TV we see women lying on their backs giv-ing birth. According to legend, and a handful of scholars such as Lauren Dundes (a professor of sociology), the start of this practice was due to King Louis XIV's fascination with watching women give birth. He had over 22 children by both wives and mistresses and found that he could see much more easily what was happening if the mother was lying on a bed rather than squatting or standing. Another source of this birthing position is credited to François Mauriceau, a French obstetrician, who wrote in 1668 that hori-zontal births were more convenient, for the doctor. He also wrote about pregnancy as an illness rather than a natural condition and in this way the influential man contributed to the medicalisation of birth.

Please know this: the female body is amazingly intelligent and wonderfully evolved for natural birth. As the pregnancy contin-ues, the relaxin hormone starts to soften the joints of the pelvis to create more room for the baby to move through. This allows movement of the usually rigid pelvis both at the front at the pubic symphysis (where the pubic bones meet) and at the back on either side of the sacrum. As the baby's head moves down, it pushes the sacrum back. This movement of the joints allows something called nutation and counter-nutation: that is, flexion to create more space as the baby's head enters the pelvis and as it leaves it. In conjunction with the baby's skull bones being able to move, this spaciousness supports the birth journey.

The natural intelligence also guides the baby into an ideal position for starting birth: head down! This ideal position for the baby to start labour is sometimes called the Optimal Foetal Position (OFP). The baby's intrinsic intelligence is supported by the mother moving *if* she feels like moving, or choosing a position that feels comfortable. This is because moving the hips moves the pelvis and this changes the space available to the baby inside. This movement might create enough space to move a little hand away from the face (and thus improve positioning for birth) or for the baby to look down so that the smallest surface area of the baby's head is available to move through the birth canal.

Movement also relaxes the mother's muscles and enables the connective tissue to glide more easily, creating as much space as possible in the expansion phase (between contractions) for the baby to move into the best position possible. An ancient sculpture from Egypt shows Cleopatra (69–30BC) kneeling down to give birth, surrounded by five attendants. There are numerous other images of women being upright in birth that have been recorded throughout history. Women's maternity notes should be branded with: if mum can move her pelvis, baby can move.

Having said that, you might feel the need to be still and rest during the birth. Lying on your left side would be ideal for this, rather than on the back, to encourage good positioning of the baby. Lying on your back creates an uphill journey for your baby over the sacrum and tailbone, whereas side-lying enables the body to move easily to accommodate the hidden journey that your baby is making of spiralling through the pelvis. For example, on your side, the pelvis is able to tilt so that the tailbone moves out of the way as the baby's head emerges for the unpoetically named 'ejection reflex', whereas lying on the back blocks this instinctive manoeuvre. Giving the body permission to respond to what is happening, rather than imposing what birth should look like, creates a ripple effect of permission deep into a woman's psyche to accept that she has all that she needs on every level.

Following are two mums tell their birthing stories where they followed the urge to move around during labour.

HESTER'S BIRTHING STORIES

(hospital birth, homebirth)

Hester is a petite woman with lots of energy and a great sense of humour. She was always so friendly in Mother and Baby Yoga classes, making sure to include those on the outside of conversations.

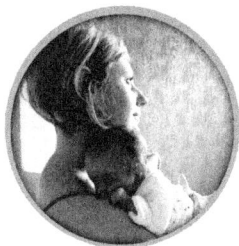

Elise's birth:

Like most first-time mums I remember being excited and terrified about going through the birthing process. I had watched a lot of 'One Born Every Minute' prior to getting pregnant: this and other births you see on telly had built up my expectations that there would be a lot of screaming and wanting to kill the father – very worrying!

Our NCT classes had provided a refresher on the biology behind birth: abstract concepts like oxytocin, contractions and epidurals.

I also did a pregnancy yoga class and found that much more useful in terms of learning practical ways to get through labour. I felt empowered that I could influence things by changing positions and understanding how my body works. However, the unknown was still the unknown. I remember thinking, "I've never

*even broken a bone before. Will it be more painful than that?"
I just had no idea what it would feel like.*

*Our plan was to give birth in the midwife-led unit (MLU), in a
birthing pool. Everyone seemed to suggest this would be the
best place, with the labour ward much more scary and likely
to end in intervention. However, with only four rooms, and stories of how busy the MLU could get, and even that the hospital
might close and we could be sent as far as Southampton, I was
anxious before we went into labour that I might not get the
option we had chosen.*

*My contractions started as mild period pains in the evening. I
knew it could be a false start ... or the start of a marathon so I
somehow managed to go to sleep as normal and put the prospect of going into labour out of my mind. In the morning the
contractions were still very mild but regular. It was a Bank Holiday and we went to my in-laws for lunch as planned. I happily
ate lunch and chatted away normally.*

*By the evening things were ramping up. At 9pm I sent my part-
ner up to bed to get some rest and swayed through the contractions as they increased in intensity whilst the telly was on in the
background (I couldn't concentrate on it). I found the pain really
hard to handle – even at this stage. I couldn't sit down or lean
forward on my birthing ball – both were excruciating, and it
really felt like there was no let up between contractions. When
one ended, the next one started almost straight away. This was
NOT what the textbooks say!*

*So I stood and breathed my calming yoga breaths and swayed
and tried to stay calm. After a while I hid myself away in the
downstairs toilet! I turned the lights out, sat down backwards
and leaned on the cistern, whilst tracking my contractions on
my phone. I had a TENS machine and got myself into the zone,
pushing the button at the height of the contractions and trying
not to think about how slowly time was ticking away. I remem-*

ber fumbling with my phone to unlock it and record the contractions accurately. The light from the phone took me out of my zone every time and I was anxiously monitoring myself to get to the magic number so that we could call triage and get to hospital. I wasn't hungry or thirsty. Just massively in pain and scared that I had no control over the contractions. They had started and I couldn't make them stop.

At around 1am my partner came down to check on me. I jumped on the chance to move things along and insisted he call the triage line. My contractions were coming every three minutes and I was anxious to get to the hospital, to the pain relief and into the pool. The hospital tried to convince me to stay at home, but they had room in the MLU and my contractions were consistently coming at the required level. I didn't want to wait and miss the room. And I REALLY wanted pain relief. So we got into the car and drove to the RBH. It's only a ten-minute journey. Somehow, we made it there without too much craziness.

When we arrived, reception was brightly lit and empty. I remember feeling really annoyed with the midwives who seemed to be patronising and not understanding the amount of pain I was in, saying things like: "I can tell that you're not in full labour yet because you're still talking". Grrrrrrr! I was grumpy and rude in a way I would never normally be. But the pain was too much. They examined me in a small, brightly lit room, with an ultrasound machine in it. When I lay down on the hospital bed, the contractions eased and slowed down for the first time since they'd become so relentless and unbearable. I was delighted. Finally, some respite. But then devastation when they told me the worst possible news: I was only 1cm dilated.

Even worse, I was massively dehydrated so they wanted to hook me up to an IV for fluids. I was in ketosis. This was why my pain was so severe. Something inside me knew I didn't want a cannula. I'd be tied to a bed and never get the birth I wanted. While we waited for the midwives to take me off, I stood in reception, swaying, swearing and downing hundreds of cups of water. It was a long wait in the barren reception in the wee small hours of the morning. Eventually we were taken down to the labour ward and into a freezing cold, tiny room, with just enough room for a bed. I lay down and the contractions and pain slowed again. I was thankful again. A new test showed I had rehydrated myself and could avoid the IV. They told me to go home. That I'd be more comfortable there. But I refused.

I wanted to stay in the cold room on the bed where the contractions eased. Going home seemed like a massively backwards step. My partner was tired and wanted to follow their advice. He knew we were nowhere near. It was here, for the first time, as he pleaded with me to go home and I pleaded with him to let me stay, that we hugged and I realised that hugging him also made the contractions less painful, more bearable. I realised I hadn't held him at all up until now. My instinct to shut myself off and deal with it alone had meant I hadn't recognised how stressed and panicky I was. I was doing my yoga breathing but minutely following the clock and the frequency of contractions. No wonder it wasn't working. It took a long time and a lovely positive midwife to finally convince me to leave. We arrived back home at 6am tired and facing the prospect of a long labour.

I got into the bath, turned out the lights and put on a meditation podcast which I played over and over. I remember the pattern of contractions coming like waves, rolling in, ramping up, then rolling away. In my zoned-out state, I understood them and came to a place where I could deal with them. I didn't want interruptions. That just brought the reality crashing back. Unfortunately, my partner, anxious to make sure I was ok, kept coming in to check I hadn't drowned. He tried to get me to eat a crumpet at one point – but it just made me sick. I remember pacing up and down the living room loudly exhaling 'Aaaaaaaaaahhh' like at a dentist, as my yoga teacher had *taught us. This terrified my partner and amused me a little. But I think it helped to channel the pain.*

Somehow, I pushed on and made it to 2pm. We again made the journey to the hospital by car. This time the traffic was worse. I felt worse. But thankfully when they examined me, I had made it to 4cm and I went straight away into a large warm bath. Out came the gas and air and I relaxed. This was it. It was happening. I felt safe and happy that the worst was over. And I was right. Things progressed much quicker from this point.

We had two midwives assigned to us: one student and one bookish type lady with glasses. I'm sad to say I don't know her name or remember much about her. I stayed in the bath for a long time enjoying the gas and air (a little too much). My partner put on the music we had selected but I couldn't say I noticed. He relayed messages to me for the midwives because I wasn't listening to them and I marvelled at how he knew what to do! I certainly relaxed in the care of midwifes and with the (long overdue) pain relief.

I stayed in one position leaning out of the bath for a long time and eventually the midwife advised me to get up and go for a wee. When I came back, they guided me to a bean bag by the window at the top of the hospital: I remember the views across Reading and being told I could try to push. Exhilarated by reaching this milestone I had new energy and focus. This is where I tried out lots of positions I'd learnt from yoga class to help the baby down. When I got to crowning stage and I felt the burn, I remembered a close friend saying she hadn't worried about it by then; she had just wanted the baby out. And that spurred me on to not to be afraid, to embrace the moment, knowing the baby was almost here. I pushed down with all my might. Just a few times.

And then she came. I was standing with one leg up on a ledge. I remember seeing her fall down, a flash of blue, that the midwife caught and took away. 17.25. I had wanted delayed cord-clamping but they took her off to help her get breathing. I wasn't scared. I was elated she was finally out! I remember shouting across the room "Is it a boy?!" I thought I heard them say it was. But it was a beautiful, tiny, long limbed blue girl with pink cheeks and a scrunched-up face. She had two large lumps on her head from the long labour pressing down on the cervix for so long. I held her and smelled her smell. We did skin-to-skin. Magical.

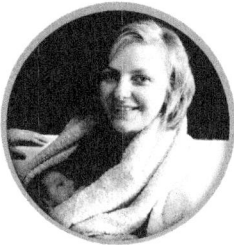

Finn's birth:

Preparing for Finn was much less intense. The only thing I did this time was to take a few pregnancy yoga classes again to help refresh my memory on what to do in labour and to watch a few of the recommended video materials including Tessa's opening flower and the wave birthing mediations [see Resources].

We had considered homebirth for our first baby. But ultimately, like many first-time parents, chose the MLU to help us in case there were any problems during the birth. Second time around, despite being a 'good candidate', and many prompts from my prenatal midwives, we chose the MLU again, as this had been a positive experience for us previously.

HOWEVER! Two weeks before due date, my other half broke his leg. Logistically, this meant much more stress getting to and from the hospital. I dreaded being sent home and having to do it all twice, as we had in my previous labour.

So, at 39 weeks, we invited the homebirth team to talk us through the homebirth option. They came armed with evidenced-based research to reassure us on the safety aspects and the possible reasons for transfer to hospital. Most of which were not emergency/scary scenarios. We had a really high chance of delivering at home without complications, I'd get gas and air (very important!) and all our postnatal appointments at home. So we felt pretty positive about changing our plans and going for a homebirth. Fortunately for us, our community midwife/very kind neighbour, lent us her pool and kit so we were all set up within a couple of days. It kind of all slotted into place.

Then my sister sent me some affirmation cards. I hadn't done hypnobirthing and I hadn't really embraced the idea of affirmations. But I pinned a few to the fridge: 'Everything is going to be okay', 'My body knows what to do', 'I look forward to meeting my baby' and I liked the tone they set. Positive rather than negative, worrying thoughts.

One of our biggest concerns had been our toddler and how we might get her off to her grandparents without too much distress. The homebirth midwife somehow managed to plant a seed in my head that some toddlers sleep through everything and that labour might be much quicker and less noisy than the first time around .... a little hope came into my thoughts .... when previously it had been dismissed as not an option.

Being at home and being my second labour meant I felt much more prepared and calmer about dealing with contractions and managing the pain. When contractions started in the middle of the night, I didn't time them or wake my other half, I tried to stay resting and not get anxious. I just lay in bed and breathed through them, reciting the 'I am calm. I am strong' affirmation from Tessa's class and using all my breathing techniques.

After a while I started to track the contractions on my phone. I tried not to get too excited when I realised that I'd reached the threshold to call the midwife. She was very calm and reassuring, put me on the system and gave me another milestone to reach before phoning again. I felt calm and excited. I visualised the waves and opening rose to get me to contractions lasting one minute every three to four minutes and called for the midwife to come.

At 7am I woke my partner and told him we were on. He got our little girl ready for nursery and I stayed out the way in our bedroom, listening to the everyday chitter chatter about getting dressed. They were jolly. I was breathing through the contractions as they got stronger. Just before they left, my little girl came into the room. She was totally oblivious to my state – she bounced around the room a bit, chatting, and I tried to not alert her to my labouring state! I crossed the room and dived into the en suite, closing the door so I could bend over and deal with the pain. They left shortly after that and I jumped straight into the bath.

I put the radio on my phone and continued my golden thread breathing whilst the pool was being set up downstairs...we didn't make it that far. I was examined at 9.30am and was so relieved to hear I'd made it to 6cm. I had been preparing myself to be told I was 1cm as I had with my first labour. So now I felt elated and even more confident in how I would birth this baby. "Gas and air, please" I joyfully requested. Then went back to the bath. The waters burst pretty quickly after that and I knew I had to push straight away. My other half reluctantly gave up his efforts to fill the pool and came up to be with me for the final stage. He massaged my back and I had a few inhalations of gas and air. After a couple of pushes Finn was born at 10.25am weighing 7lbs 6oz. He was handed straight to me for skin-to-skin and a lovely cuddle.

So second babies are quicker! And not being afraid of the contractions really made a difference for me this time. The midwife said it was the most chilled labour she had ever seen!!

Like everyone says, one of the nicest things about a homebirth is to be able to get into your bed afterwards for a cuddle and rest. The midwives look after you very gently and carefully, performing checks and bringing you tea/knickers/towels and biscuits! There are no interruptions or rules to follow like you have on a labour ward. So you really do get to relax and enjoy the moment.

I think one of the things we missed out on because of our late decision to have a homebirth, was to build a relationship with the midwife team, which lots of other people have talked about. However, our duty midwife – Jo – was amazing during our birth and came to visit us at home for almost all our follow-up appointments after birth. So now I really feel a bond with her and the team in a way I didn't get the first time around having all postnatal appointments at the hospital. I look forward to telling our son about how he came into the world and that Jo was a part of it.

In her second birthing journey, Hester moved around home finding out what positions and movements worked for her. When her daughter was bustling around, she found a cocoon of privacy in the toilet. She was aware of how her senses were heightened during labour and moved to work with them for maximum benefit.

SUE'S BIRTHING STORY

(homebirth, hospital transfer)

(Sue is a pseudonym)

Reading is half an hour from London by train and I have people from all over the world come to my classes. Sue was not fazed by being away from her home country, navigating a different maternity system and deciding what birth was right for her.

My pregnancy was amazing, I enjoyed every minute of my growing belly and the life I felt inside me. I wasn't anxious about giving birth, I was looking forward to it and I felt very prepared and calm after being to pregnancy yoga and hypno-birthing classes.

For me the most important thing was to give birth at home. I knew that I would feel more relaxed and in control. But I re-alised when it comes to childbirth you can't plan everything. When I was 41 weeks plus 2 days, I decided to have a sweep to get things (hopefully) started. My midwife told me I was al-ready 2cm dilated and I felt that it was not going to take long before we could hold our baby in our arms. That afternoon I felt like I was having period pain and I spend the rest of the day on the sofa watching Netflix and went to bed early.

At five o'clock I woke up with a feeling that my labour just start-ed. I didn't wake up my husband, to give him a bit more rest, and went downstairs for a cup of tea. I went over to the sofa and nestled up with a blanket. I timed my contractions using a labour contraction timer, they came every five minutes. I paid attention on my breathing and I imagined the contraction being like a mountain, the pain getting heavier at the top and then calming down again. After each contraction there was nothing for five minutes and I felt completely calm and relaxed.

After two hours being downstairs in my own world, I decided to wake up my husband so he could set up the pool. While he was getting the pool ready, I took a warm bath. I tried to relax my shoulders and soften my jaw, and this really helped me with relaxing my whole body. I listened to birth affirmations and when my contractions were every three minutes, I asked my husband to phone the midwife.

Both of us went downstairs and I put on some classical music. I used my pregnancy ball, walked up and down the living room and used every space in the house. I tried to keep moving around because I noticed that it helped me. Suddenly I felt like I needed to push, I felt like my body had taking over and it was very overwhelming. My husband rang the midwife again as I started to panic that we might have a baby on our own. Luckily the midwife came very quickly, and she told me I was doing very well and that I just needed to listen to my body.

I went into the pool for about 20 minutes, but it didn't give me that relaxing feeling that I had imagined. I felt like I needed to stay more active. I used the wall to lean against like I've been practicing during yoga and moved around a lot. I felt a burning sensation and I was a bit shocked by this. My midwife told me not to be scared and that it's a normal feeling. This helped me to cope. During the last bit of my labour the midwife couldn't find baby's heartbeat anymore. She wasn't panicking but called an ambulance just in case. I felt like I needed to get the baby out and that I had enough of it. The midwife told me to push actively.

And there she was ... perfectly healthy and fine. Our baby girl. I wish I could have stopped the time to let this moment sink in, but they had to check me to see if everything was okay. My hus-

band held our daughter because I didn't want her to feel that I was in pain. I used gas and air. Unfortunately, I had to go to hospital for stitches and nearly straight after giving birth both me and my daughter got dressed and went into the ambulance. She cried nearly the whole way to the hospital and I couldn't do anything about it except talk to her. That night I didn't let go of her.

I look back at a wonderful homebirth and I wouldn't change a thing. Being in my own living room with lovely music on the background made me feel so calm and relaxed. But I still feel sad about what happened afterwards. It was necessary for me to go to hospital, but for weeks I felt extremely guilty that I wasn't there for her when she needed me in the first hour of her life.

What I find most striking about Sue's story is her acceptance of a different outcome from the one she had hoped for. The sudden change of plans to go to hospital was not easy for Sue, but it did not taint the beauty of her birthing journey.

In her labour, Sue thought she would get much relief in the birth pool, but it turned out not to be what her body needed. Sometimes what we expect to help us find more comfort does not work out that way at all. With all the active birth that I teach, I had expected to be bouncing on my ball and moving rhythmically through my labours, but in fact spent the first stage both times lying down on the sofa on my left side resting and riding the surges inwardly. That is why it is crucial to have a number of options for positioning and pain relief (including different breathing techniques, TENS, water, slow movement, self-relaxation, drugs).

Attending a pregnancy yoga class helps women know the many options that are available to them during the birthing journey:

moving from this idea of lying on your back being stuck in one position, to freely being able to change between different positions. I also show women how you can use a rebozo, a South American scarf, to relax the muscles that are working so hard and take some of the weight of the baby (between contractions), or to encourage the baby to turn into a more favourable position (e.g. out of a back-to-back position). You can watch a video on how to use a scarf from the Suggestions list below.

Sometimes there can be a surge of adrenaline during the labour and then the flight or fight response can be triggered. This can result in a lot of energy being available to the arms and legs, which can feel uncomfortable and disorientating from the work of labour. In these situations, it can be helpful to hold something in your hands like stress balls or rolled up socks that you can squeeze the life out of (rather than your partner's hands!) or to stamp your feet or, if you're kneeling, kick your feet onto a pillow or mat underneath. This can also be an additional tool as contractions intensify and you need a way of releasing the powerful energy in your body. If you're lying on your side you can rub the top foot over the bottom leg, up and down repeatedly, or rub the feet together as a way of shifting your focus. Any kind of movement helps you feel that there is something you can positively do to manage the surges.

I studied belly dancing over several years and when Helen, one of my teachers, became pregnant with her second child, I asked her about the first birth. I was so curious – did she dance during the labour? She looked at me with amazement and said it didn't cross her mind. Dancing is not only her job, but her passion in life and I wondered what would have encouraged her to move. I suggested that in the second birth she might consider moving however felt good. When she went into labour the second time around, she went on to play music and sway her hips in a way that eased the contractions. Dancing can release endorphins, our natural pain-killers. Beta endorphins are stronger than morphine, so these are essential if we are to avoid or delay external forms of pain relief.

Remaining active during pregnancy is key to preparing for an active birth. One pregnant lady that attended my classes, Hilary, would arrive on her bicycle throughout pregnancy to full term. The plan was to phone their neighbour for a lift to the hospital during labour, but on the big night, the car was at the garage. Her husband rang for a taxi but they said there would be a wait of half an hour. Hilary decided she couldn't wait that long and set off on her bicycle. Every time she had a contraction she would stop and breathe deeply, then set off again. Her husband was following on his bicycle with the hospital bag. When she arrived at the maternity department, they discovered she was already 9cm dilated and birthed her baby not long after. The midwives concluded that cycling was excellent for labour! While I'm not suggesting you take up cycling if you didn't use this for transport or exercise before pregnancy, being active keeps you healthy and moving, and prepares your body for birthing.

In pregnancy yoga, we move through different postures and movements to support activity and health during the antenatal time, but we are also practicing what may help during the birth. Through this embodied practice, we can find what suits our bodies and create a body memory of what may help during the birth journey. One of many positions that allow pelvic mobility, is the squat (Box 8). Becky Reed, a UK midwife with an amazing home-birth rate, found that when women are supported to follow their instincts, they tend to choose a leaning, kneeling position for birth. This position has so many benefits: being upright enables the baby's head to rest on the cervix to support dilation, gravity helps the baby to move downwards, the pelvis is supported and free to move, whatever the mother is leaning on can be pushed against during contractions to help with the intensity, and it's easy to rest during the expansion phase.

BOX 8: Regular squatting

In every pregnancy yoga class I incorporate squats because they are beneficial in a number of ways: leg strength is important for an active birth, the squats tone the muscles around the pelvis as the joints soften, keeping the structure stable, the movement stretches the perineal tissue slightly aiding elasticity and stretch-ability, and finally they build stamina.

Stand with your feet wider than hip width (up to 50cm apart if you don't have pelvic pain) and angle the feet at 45 degrees. As you bend the knees, check that they are pointing in the same direction as your toes. Sit back so your bottom sticks out behind and you're leaning forwards with your torso. You need to be able to return out of the squat without using your hands on your legs, so build up the depth of squat over time.

First set of 3: hands on your hips, breathe out to squat down with your bottom back, breathe in to return, giving an extra squeeze to your buttocks.

Second set of 3: lift your arms towards the ceiling as you breathe out and squat down, lower your arms as you breathe in and return.

Third set of 3: hands on hips, breathe out and squat down a third of the way, then two thirds, then as low as you're comfortable to go. Breathe out to return, again in thirds.

(NB. There should not be any pain in the pelvis or hips so stop if there is. Also, if there is a feeling of heaviness within the pelvis when doing the squats, stop and seek support.)

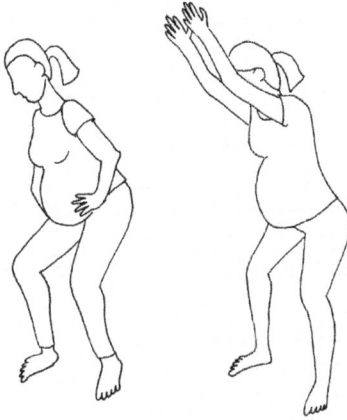

There are also certain movements that can support specific situations. A student in my class named Manuela had opted for an epidural during her labour and managed to get some rest once it set in. However, the midwife said that the baby was taking too long in this stage and wanted to get the consultant to discuss using forceps. If there was one thing that Manuela did not want, it was forceps, and so she asked her husband to help her get off the bed (this is possible with a mobile mix epidural) and onto all fours. She remembered a position from class called the Gaskin manoeuvre where you bring one leg as far forwards as you can. (This can help the baby's shoulders move through the pelvis.) At that moment the midwife and consultant appeared and shot forwards because they could see the baby's head emerging! Sometimes positioning is everything.

A note about epidurals: because of the numbing effect, there are no longer the same signals from the body to do all the things that have been helping to that point. Instead, the atmosphere will have changed; the lights go on to site the epidural, the anaesthetist starts talking you through the process, and you are more likely to start chatting, as you can no longer feel the contractions. All of this can mean that the neocortex has been activated (see Pearl 1 for why you don't want to do this) and the hormones that have been keeping your contractions coming regularly like oxytocin and melatonin may drop. If contractions become less effective, interventions like forceps and ventouse are more likely. Instead, consider turning the lights down again, asking everyone to be quiet so you can rest or focus, and be in a position that enables you to move your pelvis (like on your left side). You can write this into your birth preferences.

Your baby is not passive during the birth but will push with the legs to help move down through the birth canal and move a hand away from his or her face if given a chance. There was a Facebook post with an incredible video of a baby being born via caesarean and the surgeon gave time for the baby to push himself out through the opening in the mother's womb/tummy, at the ready in case he needed any assistance. A beautiful visualisation that I learnt from Catherine Shainberg, a psychologist and Kabbalah teacher, aids the mother's opening for dilation and can also be adapted in the case of caesarean birth. See my version in Box 9 (and reference in Resources). The golden rule is to do what makes you feel most comfortable, but if that isn't having the desired effect, **try something else**!

BOX 9: Golden oil visualisation

Ask your partner to read this out loud to you slowly or record yourself.

Sit or lie in a comfortable position. Imagine holding a glass vial of golden oil, warmed by the rays of the sun. You take out the stopper and put a drop on your tongue. Visualise it moving across your tongue and slowly down your throat. Picture it moving through your stomach, intestines and into the pelvic bowl.* Imagine the warm golden oil moving around the bony structure of the pelvis, allowing the joints to move enough to help your baby move down when the time comes. Now visualise the golden oil moving around the muscles and tissues of your pelvis, supporting the opening of the cervix to make space for your baby to come out into the world.

The golden oil also coats the amniotic sac, making it slippery. Without breaking the membranes, the oil also moves through the amniotic fluid to glide around your baby's body, making the skin glisten and your baby appear so healthy and well. Everything, your body, your baby, is slippery. The baby moves so easily down with this wonderful golden oil, down, down and out into loving waiting arms.** You picture whoever is receiving your baby having hands glistening with the golden oil, so your baby feels comforted and safe. Imagine looking into your baby's eyes. When you're ready, open your eyes.

(*Good bacteria does in fact move into the vagina to 'seed' your baby's immune and digestive systems – see microbiome references below. **This can be adapted for caesarean births so that you also imagine that there is golden oil around the incision through the belly and on the hands of all the people in the room, waiting to support the birth of your baby, doing the best job they have ever done.)

📖 REFLECTIONS) on Moving Freely

Take a moment to reflect on how you feel about moving your body in general. It may depend on a myriad of factors from personal body image and self-esteem to cultural and social messages you've received about moving your female body.

What position do you assume you will be in to birth your baby? Why?

How do you feel about active birth positions like standing, leaning over, squatting, kneeling or all fours? Do they seem primitive to you or natural? Hard work or empowering?

What would encourage you to move if you're at hospital? (E.g. Taking music with you, putting your arms around your partner's neck and swaying, leaning against the wall and moving your hips.)

Do you feel like you need permission to move in certain environments? Why?

💡 SUGGESTIONS)

Attend a pregnancy yoga class where birthing positions are included. (Some classes focus on being active and healthy during pregnancy, which is brilliant, but see if there is one available that also covers active birth.)

Create a playlist of songs that you can move to during labour.

Watch videos on how to use a rebozo for releasing back ache during pregnancy and aiding baby's position during labour. (Search for Sophie Messager Rebozo as a starting point on YouTube.)

RESOURCES

Becky Reed (2016) *Birth in Focus*, Pinter & Martin.

Catherine Shainberg (2014) *DreamBirth: Transforming the Journey of Childbirth through Imagery*. 161 Practices for Conception, Pregnancy, Labour, and Bonding. Sounds True.

www.spinningbabies.com for videos on different techniques for changing the position of your baby.

Jean Sutton and Pauline Scott (1995) *Understanding and Teaching Optimal Foetal Positioning*. Birth Concepts.

http://microbirth.com/the-film/ for insight into the role of mothers' microbes for optimal infant immune system and health.

Alexis Dunn et al. (2017) *The Maternal Infant Microbiome: Considerations for Labor and Birth*. MCN Am J Matern Child Nurs. 42(6): 318-25. (Whole article available at https://www.ncbi.nlm.nih.gov/pmc/articles/PMC5648605/)

Pearl 5
Feminine Strength

*The support of a woman
who can fully empathise is
transformative.*

Imagine there is a woman whom you feel so comfortable with that you can be totally yourself in any situation and know that you will not be judged. That during birth you can do whatever makes you comfortable and she will be there making everything easier. You know that she has given birth and understands the depths of the inner resources that you need to call on. She knows when to give you space and when to stroke your hair: she is full of empathy.

We're so far from the matriarchy of times gone past that it can be difficult to understand what feminine power looks like. Although we may have women breaking glass ceilings at work, it is still very much in a masculine environment and there are few role models for feminine leadership. One example may be Jacinda Ardern, Prime Minister of New Zealand, who openly cried after the mosque shootings in 2019 and was praised for showing deep compassion. That this emotionally open leadership is so unusual is troubling. Another role model is Clare Dubois of the TreeSisters charity, who aims to lead from an authentic feminine stance; being guided by intuition as well as the head, and giving employees time off during their menstruation to rest.

In mainstream education, intuition is something not to be nurtured but actively scorned. In school we are usually taught to write "I think" rather than "I feel" because we will be taken more seriously. In academia articles are written in the third person, distancing even further the author from the idea. However, women-centred midwives use their intuition and empathy to understand what part of a birth journey a labouring woman has reached, alongside cues from her body such as a change in her voice, the temperature of her legs, the purple line across the sacrum. Parents use their gut feeling to seek help when something is seriously wrong with a child who is ill but is not old enough to explain how they feel or what is wrong.

Feminine strength can look very different from mainstream ideas of strength and power. For example, being strong might be using intuition to know when to wait and when to forge ahead. It may be a companion who shows great empathy in providing individual-ised support and honouring a woman's preferences, although the birth may not be progressing in a 'text-book' way. Female strength may be trusting the necessity to yield and being alright with *being* in labour rather than 'doing birth'. Men can tap into these femi-nine strengths of course and there are excellent male midwives, but perhaps there is nothing like a person who has given birth to totally support you from an embodied knowledge of birthing.

Here are two mums talking about how they were supported by the Feminine.

JOEY'S BIRTHING STORY

(hospital birth, supported by sisters)

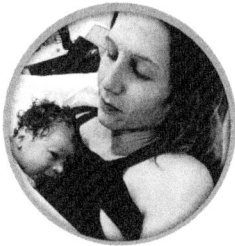

Esmae's birth:

I woke up about 3am with a real need for a cup of tea and some biscuits! This is not something that I ever do so it was very out of character – but, as always, I followed what my body wanted and went down and got my biscuits! I popped to the toilet before I got back into bed (with the tea and biscuits) and noticed I had a very light pink discharge. I had a very slight dull ache in my tummy, which at first I possibly mistook for hunger but actually began to feel more like a very mild period pain. I went back to sleep and woke a few more times – my 'period pain' continuing but it was of no discomfort.

When I woke at about 7.30am I rang the hospital to tell them of my symptoms (I was 1 day overdue and as it had been previously discovered that I was a Strep B carrier, I had been told to ring them as soon as I had signs). They alarmed me a little by telling me that the hospital had actually stopped admitting patients and instead had been sending them to other hospitals – although they reassured me that by the time I would need to be in they would probably be admitting patients again! Then I sent a message to my family – who live in Somerset – to inform them. My sisters told me they would do the school run and then drive straight up to me! I messaged a close friend who lives nearby and told her that I was fine but to be on standby in case things happened really quickly!

My morning was spent mainly eating and drinking and watching tv on my yoga ball. Interestingly I never used my yoga ball during pregnancy – but when it came to my contractions it was the only thing that I wanted!!! I also double checked that I had my bags packed and messaged my baby's father so that he was aware of what was happening.

Both of my sisters arrived, and we had lots of rounds of (decaf) tea and sandwiches. I discovered that if I sat on my yoga ball (my safe place), then my contractions calmed down and slowed down! My sisters reminded me that this WASN'T what I wanted and so I remained very mobile, walking around the house. But as soon as I got a contraction, I practically ran to my yoga ball to help ease through the contraction.

It was wonderful having my sisters focus on the timings of the contractions and I just focused on my body and its needs (which included a lot of toilet trips! I'm not sure if my body was nervous or just clearing out!!!)

Eventually the hospital agreed that we should go in (they were admitting patients again!) and so we piled everything into the car and went in. I found the car journey difficult as it wasn't very spacious and the difficulty with parking was not appreciated!!!! I think I would have started to panic a little at this point but then I remembered Tessa talking about the possible difficulty of the journey to the hospital so I made myself as comfortable as possible and reminded myself that the time would pass! During my pregnancy I collected a number of quotes about giving birth and I really focused on these during the more difficult moments.

Once I was at the hospital we got taken through to a room where one midwife suggested I was about ready to have a room whilst the other disagreed saying there wasn't any room yet! (Unfortunately, the birthing centre was closed due to such high numbers of patients.) None of this fazed me and I was quite content just chatting and joking with my sisters. It was at this point that my sister suggested I try the TENS machine. I hadn't really thought about using it but my sister had brought hers, and so I had packed it into the bag without much thought. This actually turned out to be amazing for me!!! (Along with the birthing ball which I also brought with me.)

At no point in the birthing process did I focus on timings of contractions or how dilated I was...this was something that my sisters calculated for the hospital (as this appeared to be the main thing they focused on), but it was not a focus for me at all. I was just keen to keep the contractions flowing and to follow what my body wanted.

The decision was finally made that I should go home and come back in later. My sister told me that we wouldn't go home, but instead suggested that we stayed in the hospital somewhere. I agreed as I didn't want to get back in the car! I later found out that my sister said this as my mother had informed her that we are quite prone to having babies fast and she was worried we wouldn't make it back in time!!! She didn't tell me at the time in case it worried me or got my hopes up. It was so lovely having the sensitivity, thoughtfulness and kindness that only a woman can bring!

We decided to set up home in one of the hospital cafes. I sat on my birthing ball with my TENS machine on and I enjoyed a lovely dinner of jacket potato, cheese and beans!!! During this time my sister kept track of my contractions (the hospital had informed us as to when we should go back in relation to contractions – again this was not something I cared about! But thankfully my sisters were on this!) Within half an hour my contractions had met the hospital's threshold! So I went back to the ward and waited to be reas-

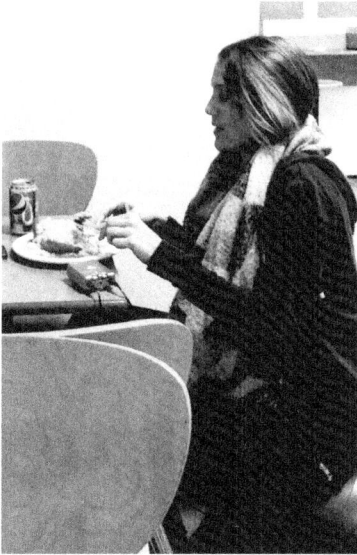

Spot the TENS machine in the above photo

sessed. At this point my contractions were getting painful and in hindsight I wish I had reached out for support/pain relief a little earlier. Just before 7pm I was given a room and given the antibiotics for strep B and also started on gas and air. I had a very open mind when it came to giving birth and knew I would just need to go with what felt right at the time – which was surprisingly being on the hospital bed. I found it most comfortable to be on all fours on the bed.

My main comfort was my music. I had my Bob Marley album on for the entire time! And every time the music stopped I became panicked until my sister restarted it! It truly helped me to be in the zone and the midwife even joked with us about how I was literally pushing and moving in time to the music!

I felt so prepared for giving birth and I put this down to the yoga classes that I did with Tessa as well as the books I read and the quotes I collected over the months of being pregnant. I was so focused on my breathing and on the music that was playing – I feel lucky that I remember every single moment of the birth – I can remember every conversation and every single thing that happened. Which, talking to others, seems quite rare!

I was so surprised at how fast it was all happening. I feel that people overemphasise how long a first birth can be...I was expecting my contractions to slow down at some point but there was literally no slowing down at any point! The midwife *couldn't believe I asked for a break so I could have a snack!!! I had brought snacks. But there was no time for snacks.*

It wasn't long before I was told I needed to start pushing. And this wasn't something that I felt prepared for. I was so confident with my breathing and in keeping my jaw relaxed so that my cervix was relaxed, etc. that I actually had no idea about pushing. The midwife banned me from the gas and air at this point because I was still 'breathing through it' when I was meant to be pushing! I didn't understand what she wanted from me until my sister whispered in my ear, "Push like you are doing a giant poo!!!" And as soon as she said that I understood and I very quickly pushed my baby into the world. I remember the midwife saying, "I can see hair – she's on her way!!" Baby Esmae was born at 10.30pm.

As soon as the midwife put my baby into my arms, I asked to have my phone, and I video called the dad. He was asking me how heavy the baby was and the midwife explained she was still joined to me. It was so important to me that he was one of the first people to 'see' the baby. The midwife had asked me about my decision regarding birthing partners and I explained to her that my partner had not been supportive of my decision to keep my baby and that he had shown very little care for me whilst I was pregnant.

I knew that giving birth would be the biggest moment in my life: the best but also the hardest and I knew I needed strong and reliable support around me. I also explained that it was important to me that everybody in the room was 100% committed to both myself and the baby – I needed to have the positive energy to get me through the birth process. As the baby's father he has rights to the baby...but not to me and my body and my birthing experience. Ideally, I would have liked him to come in as soon as the baby was born/in my arms however it all happened far too quick!

Once my baby was in my arms, I had the injection to birth my placenta a little quicker. This wasn't something that I thought I would choose, however when I was in the moment I actually just felt that my body was so tired it just wanted it over with.

One thing that I really struggled with, with giving birth, was the gore!!! I am naturally quite a squeamish person and I really disliked not knowing what was happening! When I was pushing, I kept feeling things moving and I kept asking what was happening as I really didn't like my body doing things that I didn't know about.

What was wonderful was my sisters' knowledge of this and also with their previous experience they were not fazed at all. My sister helped me afterwards to shower and even removed some of the sheets, so I didn't have to see so much of the mess.

It was so wonderful having both my sisters with me who between them have birthed five children. They truly understood how I was feeling and what needed to be done and they kept reassuring me that they had done it so therefore I could also do it – they were so supportive. In hindsight I feel it was really lovely to have BOTH my sisters as they were able to support each other too – I imagine it would feel very pressured to be the sole support, but they were also able to support each other. My sisters absolutely loved being there and one of my sisters kept announcing how broody it was making her feel! They both watched as my baby was born and one of my sisters cut the cord.

After a round of tea and toast I was taken to the ward and my sisters settled me in and then left to get some sleep before visiting time the next day. Then I gazed into my baby's eyes and remained like that for the whole night! A member of staff on the ward came round and told me I should put her down and get some rest, but I refused. I knew I would never get this night back – just me and my newborn baby...

Joey's story touches me every time I read it because her sisters were so ably attentive to her needs. Joey was able to relax into the cocoon of love and attention that they created. I love that her sisters, knowing the way that they had laboured, took her to the hospital café for baked potato rather than risk an uncomfortable journey back home.

This female support reminds me of a friend of mine whom I knew from a meditation centre that I attended in London for many years. Kirtan (singing mantras) was a beautiful practice that was usually used as a preparation for meditation. She had invited a number of us around to her home for a Mother Blessing. During the afternoon the surges began and soon became so strong that she needed to focus through each one. She wanted us to stay but needed the privacy of being in a different space so that she could concentrate with only her husband and midwife present. We sang kirtan in the next-door room continuously until we heard the baby cry, and then sang louder and sweeter than ever before. Having all of your female friends in the room next door may not be every-body's ideal support, but for her it provided spiritual strength like nothing else: everyone had one-pointed focus on the safe arrival of baby and the transition of our friend into a mother.

LIZ'S BIRTHING STORY

(epidural, episiotomy)

Liz is in a same-sex relationship and tells it like it is. She is open about her experiences and this has led to her co-hosting a local mums' group to support honest talk.

Noah's birth:

As two women, we never had the option of getting pregnant 'naturally'. The problem with not being able to just 'get on with it', means that you tend to overthink the whole thing into oblivion. So, we spent a long time researching options, talking, hypothesising and going to meet with people.

The IVF route was our preferred option, but, in reality, the cost and the prospect of large quantities of drugs when I might be perfectly capable of conceiving naturally seemed too much. The consultant we saw was remarkably unhelpful. The solicitor we saw, to draw up an agreement between us and our friend who kindly offered to help us out as a donor, was incredible, thoughtful, knowledgeable and experienced in conception with same sex couples.

We went to NCT classes and the facilitator was really proactive, corrected herself when she said, "Mums on this side of the room, and dads on the other", and allowed my partner to choose where she stood. The other couples in the class were great and we forged good friendships. We were all in the same boat, same anxieties, same questions, same needs.

We were lucky and it only took a few tries. We were also lucky because we didn't experience any discrimination, judgement or even raised eyebrows from medical professionals, antenatal care providers, or pregnancy yoga teachers. We did get some extremely inappropriate questions from acquaintances and work colleagues though. I could write a book about those!

I went into spontaneous labour at about 4am on Tuesday 14th March and Arlo arrived safely in the evening of Wednesday 15th. The birth was, in hindsight, fairly textbook. I spent the daytime on Tuesday at home, watched a film, tried to relax and rest as the contractions gradually built. By the time they were close together and felt very strong, we called the hospital and they told us to come in.

Being in the car in labour was horrible, but at least it was 1am on Wednesday and there was no traffic at all! They examined me and found I was only 1cm dilated. So disappointed, mostly about having to get back in the car, I came home, got in the bath and called again at 8am when the contractions were much, much stronger. Back we went, and this time I was a whopping 1.5cm dilated. I was desperate to be in a birthing pool, knowing that the water would ease the pain and begged to stay. And they let me use the pool, but being a high-risk patient (which I only discovered when already in labour, that's a different story), I wasn't allowed to deliver in the water.

Being in the pool was amazing, and I suddenly felt myself switch from a mentality of 'I can't do this', to saying out loud, "I can do this", over and over again. Unfortunately, I was made to get out of the pool, for fear I might deliver in there. Once out of the pool, a good four hours later, I was still only 3cm. By this point

I was starting to think there was no way I could endure this. I thought that at this rate of dilation, I'd be in labour for at least a month.

I asked for an epidural. I wish I hadn't, because what I didn't know was that I was very near the end. If I'd known that it was a possibility I would go from 3 to 10 cm in about two hours, I wouldn't have asked for all the pain medication and spent twenty minutes having a horrendous and totally pointless epidural only to deliver about 30 minutes later!

Unfortunately, we had a horrible experience with one midwife who didn't listen to me, told me I wasn't even in labour (an hour before delivery), who only used dilation and no other observations to measure progress, and left me feeling out of control and forced into decisions I didn't want to make. Thank goodness for shift changes, because the midwife team who actually delivered my little boy were amazing. I wish I'd known I could ask for a different midwife. It would have changed the entire experience for me.

Arlo arrived safely, with only a small episiotomy needed, weighing 6lbs 10 and already cuddly and bright eyed.

My partner would say that there is always a slight feeling of disempowerment or being slightly on the side-lines with the whole process, she is just the 'other mother'; there isn't a proper name for her or her role. You do have to explain who the other woman in the room is, and our relationship, every single time you see a new doctor, midwife, nurse, health visitor, etc. Every single time. But you learn a script and you reel it off and it's a tiny moment in an otherwise incredible rollercoaster of a journey.

I set up a free, inclusive, peer-to-peer support group for mums, www.becomingmums.com, with a friend I met at Tessa's Active Birth class. We both wanted a space to talk about our experiences and journeys as mothers. Since then I've met hundreds of mums, some single mums, some heterosexual mums in relationships, some gay mums, some queer mums and even a trans mum. We are continually shocked by how similar our stories all are. We are united by the journey, and we all have our differences, but there is far more that we all have in common.

If I could give any advice to other same sex families, it's not to allow anything, your sexual orientation, your skin colour, your physical ability, size, age, anything, to make you feel you don't have a voice. You are entitled to demand the best possible care and so is your partner.

Liz's story illustrates how the ability of the midwives or other health professionals to empathise with you is crucial in creating a connection. Increasingly through social media, mums are connecting to share honest conversations about how it is to mother in our current culture. In our society we often live in nuclear families, separated and perhaps many miles away from the rest of our families. There is the African proverb that it takes a village to raise a child, but the same can be true of birth. How much stronger would you feel to truly know in your heart that there is a whole community wishing you well on your journey and waiting to help you in whatever way needed?

I facilitate Mother Blessings and these are a wonderful opportunity to bring together this community. The gathering may include family members and old friends, but often is created from new friends found during pregnancy, and the support can be just as strong. My favourite part of the gathering is the Red Thread ceremony. This is usually towards the end when there has been lots of sharing of stories and affection for the mum-to-be. One red thread is passed around the circle, circling the wrists (or ankles sometimes if it would be problematic for work) of all the people there. For a moment all are connected by the thread and the intention to support the woman into motherhood. Then the thread is cut in between each person and tied off to create a bracelet. Until the baby has arrived, the thread around our wrists reminds us all of the mother and her baby, and to keep them in our hearts.

However, it might be that we just need one female supporter to make a huge difference. This may be a close friend, your sister, your mum, a doula or independent midwife that you get to know and trust. What I've noticed from discussions at the end of class is that when a woman is pregnant with a subsequent baby, a pressing question in the third trimester is about how the existing child(ren) will be cared for during the birthing journey. Often, I hear that the woman does not want her mother around during labour, even if in another room caring for the child(ren). The reason is often that she would not able to relax, with perhaps underlying reasons of a fear of judgement, intrusion, interruption or sharing too intimate an experience.

The relationship with our mother is unique because it began with a fusion of our two bodies together. Deficits in that primary relationship naturally get projected outwards onto other people or situations. In the case of a deficit, we can consciously work to fill that gap of nurturing from within ourselves rather than unconsciously seeking it from others. If you recognise that you have a 'mother wound' to some degree (see Bethany Webster in the Resources), it is valuable to reflect on these feelings because they might emerge in relation to the midwife you're assigned or as you begin to mother your own children. Then it is even more important that there is someone, whether your birth partner or someone else, whom you totally trust and with whom you can be yourself so that they can provide a container of safety for you.

One of the ways of working with the Reflections in this book is to have a listening partnership (Box 10) where you can share your thoughts and discoveries with a trusted person. Find those people who value your needs and know that it's not selfish, but actually essential, to ask for exactly the support that you need for the rite of passage of birth. For example, having someone holding your hand who really believes in you and in the naturalness of birth can make all the difference. A student midwife can be excellent in this role because they do not have the same pressures as the midwife to keep track of everything and can focus purely on emotional support.

BOX 10: Listening partnership

I have had a listening partnership with a woman I met on a course for four years. Every Tuesday we have 15 minutes each to talk about our menstrual cycle. I have learnt so much from listening to her, as well as having the space to talk and really be listened to myself. The depth of my understanding about the patterns of thoughts and behaviours throughout my cycle is largely due to this technique.

Find someone who is willing to commit to a weekly practice for a set amount of time on a topic that you have in common (e.g. someone who is approximately the same number of weeks pregnant as you or a friend who is open to exploring feelings about pregnancy and birth), is committed to talking weekly until the first one gives birth and has 20–30 minutes each week free at a specified time.

In the first half (let's say 10 minutes), one person speaks without interruption. The other person may say "Aha", "Oh yes" or "Mmm" to show they are listening but does not interject in the way that you would do in a normal conversation. (That is, "Oh that happened to me too", "I'd do this...." or "I know who you can ask about that".) It is deep listening without the need to fix, find solutions or put your own point of view across. At the end of the 10 minutes, you can ask a mundane question to bring the person back to this moment like "What colour socks are you wearing?"

You then swap over, the listener becomes the talker and vice versa. It's fine to have times of silence: they don't need to be filled, listening to the silence and the hesitation is part of it. At the end, again ask a mundane question to bring the person back to the present like "What did you eat for breakfast?" Then you can say goodbye and hang up the call. If you both agree, you can offer some suggestions, but that is not part of the listening partnership per se. For example, my friend is a homeopath and so sometimes I will ask for her advice on a relevant remedy given what I've talked about during my turn.

REFLECTIONS on Feminine Strength

This section is about our relationship to the feminine: there may be a different question not listed below that calls for your reflection.

Do you trust your intuition, or have you learnt to override it? How could you start listening to your gut or womb again? (E.g. Noticing when you override a feeling that you can't explain.)

Write about how you feel supported or not in this transition to motherhood (again). How could you increase the support around you? (E.g. Can you ask friends or family explicitly for help? Could you join a Red Tent during pregnancy or hire a doula?)

What are your relationships with other women like? (E.g. Are you able to be yourself utterly and completely? What stops you feeling free to be yourself?)

Out of the women you know, who would you choose to be your female birth support? What qualities do they have? What stops you from having that person at the birth?

Journal about the mother you needed as a child, the mother you need now and may not have. How can you mother yourself?

💡 SUGGESTIONS

Consider having a Mother Blessing to feel and gather the support from your female friends and family. You can create your own or ask someone to facilitate it for you.

Attend a Red Tent or other women's circle where the space is held so that women can really listen to each other.

Create a Listening Partnership with another pregnant woman or someone who has been pregnant so that you are regularly held. If you need emotional support, self-refer to Talking Therapies or consider Hypnotherapy for specific anxieties about birth that your intuition is telling you are important for how your birth unfolds.

🔍 RESOURCES

Anita Diamant (1997) *Red Tent*. Wyatt Books.

https://redtentdirectory.com

Amy Wright Glenn (2013) *Birth, Breath, & Death: Meditations on Motherhood, Chaplaincy, and Life as a Doula*. Createspace.

Bethany Webster (2020) *Discovering the Inner Mother: A Guide to Healing the Mother Wound and Claiming Your Personal Power*. William Morrow.

115

Natalie Meddings (2017) *How to Have a Baby: Mother-Gathered Guidance on Birth and New Babies*. Eynham Press.

Jackie Singer (2009) *Birthrites: Rituals and Celebrations for the Child-bearing Years*. Permanent Publications.

www.handinhandparenting.org (Further information on listening partnerships.)

www.positivebirthmovement.org (Often run by doulas or other birth professionals and a good source of feminine wisdom!)

Pearl 6
Discernment

You matter. Your body, your ideas,
your intuitions, your expectations,
your decisions matter.

Imagine that as you move through the birthing journey, the midwife asks how you would like to approach each part and gently provides the expertise she has gained from assisting so many births before. Mostly she is in the background, only coming into your field of awareness when you want guidance. She is hands off, unless you ask her to be hands on.

Over the past decades, birth has become more medicalised. The rates of inductions and caesareans are increasing, and this is not because women's bodies have dramatically changed in the last fifty years. As birth moved into hospital, it became a risk rather than a natural process and this has affected how labour is managed. When you enter a healthcare system with a myriad of policies and recommendations that control how a midwife or doctor will clinically assess your labour, the more you need to reflect on self-ownership and body sovereignty. The UK is a pioneer in many aspects of woman-centred maternity care, such as supporting standalone midwife-led units and providing homebirth services, but most birth professionals would agree that there is no room for complacency!

Throughout history, men have taken control of women's bodies and this power imbalance can be subconsciously re-enacted by health professionals, regardless of their gender. Fundamentally, this is a question of who gets to touch your body and how. The moral right of a person to have bodily integrity and control of what happens to one's own body is at the core of consent. This is more complex during pregnancy and birth because there is also the baby's body to be considered and kept safe. However, this absolutely does not negate consent around the mother's body in all its guises, including permission for something to happen, respect, clarity about a person's responses to a question, responsiveness to changing feelings, trusting autonomy, and non-entitlement over others' bodies. The book *The Roar Behind the Silence* speaks about the tension felt by professionals balancing patients' needs and their employers' demands. Most of the time, couples travelling through maternity care are thankfully oblivious to how their health professionals are doing an exceptional job in a stressful environment. Nevertheless, they need to speak up if compassion and consent slip down the list of priorities.

Often it is simply a question of having enough information to feel informed and be able to fully give consent. While an intervention may be routine for a health professional, it may be the first time you have ever considered it and so you are entitled to have comprehensive information so that you properly understand the risks and benefits of a given procedure. For example, a classic risk that is told to expectant parents is that the risk of infection doubles twenty-four hours after the membranes (waters) breaking. This is the relative risk, but the absolute risk is that the risk increases from 0.05% to 1%. The actual numbers may affect the outcome of your decision-making process. If your assigned health professional does not know the absolute risk, ask them to find out or to speak to someone who does know. This will enable you to give informed consent. While you may have total trust in doctors' clinical expertise, knowing why something is being done supports your physical and psychological integrity even if the outcome is not as hoped for (e.g. an epidural that does not have the desired effect). Or to put it another way, you went in with your eyes open.

The following story shows how the mother's eyes were closed when she approached the birth of her first son, but fully open for the second.

119

ANNA'S BIRTHING STORIES
(induced, natural, postnatal depression)

Anna is a dark-haired, dark-eyed beautiful woman who has lived in a number of countries. She describes how postnatal depression can happen regardless of the kind of birth experience.

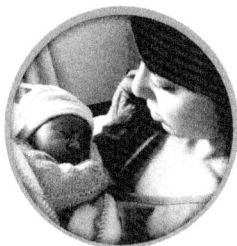

Leon's birth:

I had just travelled on my own from Italy to Bolivia while heavily pregnant. Landed, at 4080 metres above sea level, in the highest city in the world. The altitude didn't seem to have any effects on me. The new apartment was big and full of sunshine. A friend had suggested a young gynaecologist, who spoke English, because my Spanish was still basic. We had talked about my birth plan and we seemed on the same page. I was ready to start my family. I even honestly thought the hard part was over. Aha.

My waters broke two days before my due date, around 9pm La Paz time. We called the doctor and he told us to make our way to the clinic where I was going to give birth. We lived relatively far from the clinic and it made sense to drive up now that there was no traffic, rather than wait for active labour at home. "Do you have any contractions?" my husband kept asking, who

*seemed very eager to start timing them. "Not yet. I don't think".
We got to the clinic, they gave me a room and the doctor came
in. "Everything seems good", he said after examining me and
left. A nurse came in and stuck a needle in my arm. I looked at
her and she smiled. "It's a "suerito" [a serum], it's going to help
you".*

*Very shortly afterwards I started having contractions. Or what
felt like one very long, extremely painful contraction. My husband was excited to be finally useful. "Is it over? Tell me when
it's over." It never seemed to stop. And when it finally did, a
new one started right away. My husband was confused. I was
confused. Time went by, the pain was so strong it made me sick.
When the doctor finally came back, I was in tears. He seemed
annoyed. "It's called 'labour' for a reason. It's supposed to
hurt". I asked what medication they were injecting me and he
said it was Oxytocin. "To speed up the process". I asked to have
the needle removed from my arm, but the contractions didn't
stop, so I asked for an epidural and he said I couldn't get one
until I was 3cm dilated.*

*More time passed and the doctor came back. He examined me
again and said I still hadn't reached 3cm. So, once again, he
decided to "Speed up the process" and help me dilate. Using
his arm. I screamed. When the aesthetician came for the epidural the pain was so strong I was shaking. I don't remember
feeling the needle going into my spine, but I do remember the
sudden relief that followed. Finally, it was bearable. I got to rest
for a little bit and then they moved us to the delivery room.
I was exhausted. "Push!", yelled the doctor. But I couldn't really feel the contractions anymore so I just tried to guess and
pushed as hard as I could with the little energy I had left. But it
was not enough. "The baby is stuck. You need a c-section", he
announced at some point and picked up the phone to call the
surgeon.*

Then he seemed to remember I didn't want a c-section unless necessary and decided to try with the forceps first. It felt like all my organs were being pulled out of me. And then finally a cry. Leon. As soon as I saw him, I could immediately tell he looked like me.

This was not how I pictured my son's birth. None of it reflected my birth plan. Sure, in the end everything went fine. Leon was fine. I was fine. Or was I? In the following weeks I felt like I was living under a black cloud. Thankfully I had a lot of help and a wonderful paediatrician, who kept telling me I was doing a great job. So one day the black cloud went away and I didn't think about it again, until it came back until about 4 years later, when my second son was born.

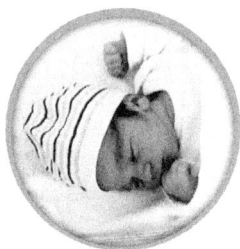

Sebastian's birth:

Sebastian was born in Reading on the 24th of October, just before midnight at 38 weeks and five days. Around lunch time that day I decided to go for a walk with my father. We walked all the way from Caversham to Reading town centre, had lunch, did some shopping and then decided to stop for coffee. Just outside of the coffee place, on Broad Street, I heard "pop" and felt warm water running down my legs. I called my husband, who came to pick me up and we drove to the hospital. After checking me, they decided I could go back home. I was only 1cm dilated and had no contractions yet.

I got home, took a bath, played with Leon and even managed to close my eyes for a bit. At around five I started feeling some very light contractions, then about an hour later some stron-

ger ones, about 10 minutes apart. I tried all of the positions we had learned during yoga and found it particularly useful to stand up against the wall. The pain was manageable until about 9pm, when I started having stronger contractions every three minutes. So I called the hospital. Apparently, because of the full moon, the population of Reading was about to double that night. As a result, the Rushey [midwife-led] clinic was full and I was asked to go to the maternity ward.

I waited at home a bit more, then at about 10pm we got to the hospital. I was expecting to spend several hours there, but things moved very quickly from that point on and Sebastian was born after only a few pushes at 11.50pm. The next day we were home. I couldn't believe how smoothly and quickly everything had gone. I was relieved and angry at the same time because I now knew how things could have been with my first birth if I hadn't been given unnecessary medication.

My body recovered easily. I lost most of the weight I had gained within a couple of weeks. We already knew how to care for a baby, so we naturally fell into a new routine and quickly forgot how life had been before. I was so pleased with myself I started filling my days with chores and activities.

Until one night I couldn't go to sleep. I was worried because Sebastian seemed to have trouble sleeping lying on his back and the GP had been very dismissive about it. "It's probably a cold. Give him paracetamol". "He's 6 weeks old". "Oh right, then just wait it out". I spent the night on the Internet and figured out that the most likely explanation was that he had reflux. The next few nights, I was up every hour, checking that Sebastian wasn't chocking on his own vomit. During the day I just kept running around as usual trying to keep up with everything.

The days were getting shorter and shorter, Christmas was coming, we were expecting guests, Leon's school had so many activities planned that I started sending myself messages during the day to keep up with all of them. At night I would awake in panic and write something down on my phone. I started realising that something was wrong when I woke up in tears one morning. The black cloud was back. I felt exhausted and trapped. I felt like I was stuck in an endless swamp. I went back to the GP. She was dismissive once again. Sent me home with a mild sleeping pill, which made me so drowsy I had a hard time waking up to breastfeed, which made me even more worried and unable to rest.

From then on things got much worse. I could feel my heart pounding every time I tried to relax. I felt I had to be everywhere at all times. No one understood what was going on. Why I wasn't sleeping? Why was I barely eating? Why was I so irritable? Ordinary things seemed impossible to bear. One afternoon I had enough. I went to a friend and asked her to drive me to the hospital. I waited in a small room for hours thinking I had gone crazy and belonged in a mad house. Sebastian was in my arms sleeping peacefully. Finally, a mental health specialist came and talked to me. They kept us the night for observation and another person came to talk to me in the morning. Postnatal anxiety was the diagnosis. I started taking antidepressants and within a few days I felt better. I started sleeping again. I felt like myself again. I realised it doesn't have to be this difficult. I was not fine and it was not "normal" to feel that way. I started enjoying life again, letting go of what was not important and giving myself time to rest and recover.

My two very different experiences taught me that maternal care is often flawed. Both during and after birth. If you are reading this and recognise yourself in any of the symptoms I described above, seek help. Make them listen, because it's not supposed to feel like this. Black clouds sometimes come, but they should go away too.

While I want this book to be a predominantly positive read, it's important to share the reality of birth within the context of the health care system globally. Many of the women in my classes are not from the UK and bring different narratives about birth from all over the world. In the vast majority of cases, it is the system which lets women down rather than the individual professionals caring for you. There are a range of reasons why maternity care across different countries can fail women: from increasing fear of litigation to stress because of under-resourced departments.

Sometimes I receive a birth story and I know that the mother physically and emotionally prepared as well as she could through various classes and courses, but that it was the external environment that derailed the birth journey. Anna's first birth story highlights this possibility so clearly. However, by reading about how natural birth physiologically happens and also about the possible interventions that may be needed, you create a knowledge bank that will give you a head start in feeling empowered to get the information you need and truly giving informed consent. Sharing birth stories is a powerful way to learn.

I remember a midwife I knew in Bristol who said that she could tell if someone had done something like pregnancy yoga. The labouring woman would walk into the room where she would birth her baby and look around, observing what was there that would help her, like a birth ball or mats on the floor, and she would get on with making herself comfortable. A woman who hadn't done a movement-based birth preparation would often arrive and stand, waiting for instruction. While it's possible for the second woman to have a wonderful birth, the midwife said that it was like starting from zero and she would need to give a lot more input. This is not ideal when you want to keep the neocortex quiet (remember Pearl

1) and follow your own instincts.

I've asked midwives what the most useful thing is to read on a birth plan (Box 11) and the answer was the woman's approach to pain relief. It might be that if you are offered pain relief, you might come to the conclusion, "She thinks I'm not coping well" and be dispirited. Alternatively, it might be that if you are not offered pain relief, you will think, "Although I'm in pain, she thinks I should be coping with it," and feel bad about asking for the pain relief available. If you can share your experience of pain and approach to pain relief, the midwife can choose her language carefully to empower you.

BOX 11: Creating your Birth Preferences

In the birth preparation workshops that I run, I ask couples to create a document with their birth preferences. This exercise usually generates a lot of questions and helps the couple to be 'on the same page' when starting the birth journey. You can download two templates from the online course (www.pearlsofbirthwisdom.com). Spend as much time thinking and writing down your ideas as you want, researching anything that you don't understand from websites such as www.aims.org.uk.

My top tips from having seen LOTS of birth plans are:

- Dream about what your ideal birth would be like (you won't jinx it!).

- Using other templates as a basis, find the words to describe what is most likely to support you to feel safe in this ideal scenario.

- Then think about the 'what ifs': what if an induction, epidural or caesarean birth were being talked about? What would your wishes be then? Write down your plan B, C, D....

- Share this process with your birth partner and gather information so you both feel more confident in your choices. It is the *process* of creating the document that is key.

- Summarise the most important points in 6–8 bullet points in a document to hand to your midwife. Remember that you are not tied to what you've written and can change your mind at any point.

- Once this process has been completed, focus on your ideal birth when visualising and daydreaming.

When athletes are preparing for a race, they visualise how they will feel when they cross the finishing line. They do not focus on losing. It sounds absurd to suggest that, so why do we discourage women from using positive psychology to prepare for birth? Mental preparation works.

I love to receive the birth stories from my clients, but I feel so sad when I read the words "I wasn't allowed to....". Finding the right language to communicate options is such an important skill, as is making time to answer questions fully in a time-watched environment. Women, their bodies and their labouring process can be fully respected when informed consent is obtained, the reasons for an intervention have been clearly communicated and the parents have given their permission to proceed. Occasionally I hear from parents that they felt emotionally coerced into a decision: this is not fair and does not lead to informed consent.

The social engagement system is frequently a missing piece of the story when people talk about the nervous system. Part of what we instinctively do as humans (and animals) is to scan for belonging.

In a healthy community, we work with others against a common threat, which in turn provides safety. Under stress we have four options: fight, flight, freeze *or* appease. As women we are apparently more likely to use appeasement because of the oestrogen hormone, which is in part about bonding. We may also decide deference is a safer option: better the threat that we can see, than the one we cannot (those hypothetical situations we're worried about). This is important because if we're feeling vulnerable, we may acquiesce our desires and choices, and may need moral support to advocate for ourselves.

Using the BRAINS acronym (Benefits, Risk, Alternative, Indication or Intuition, Nothing, Smile) to gather all the information you need can be done calmly (Box 12). In the majority of situations there is time to discuss what you have found out, just your partner and yourself, if that helps you come to a decision more comfortably. Or time to just hug and let the new situation sink in. When health professionals meet your need for this information, your feeling of safety skyrockets and the mother comes out of the experience feeling that her integrity has been respected, like in the next story.

BOX 12: Use your BRAINS

Benefits – What are the benefits of this intervention?

Risk – What is the absolute risk of proceeding with this intervention? (Remember the absolute risk is the actual numbers rather than a proportion or percentage given for the relative risk.)

Alternative – Is there an alternative course of action in this situation? What are the benefits and risks of the alternatives?

Indication/Intuition – What is the clinical indication here, based on their clinical knowledge and experience? What is your intuition or gut feeling telling you about what to do?

Nothing – What if you do nothing for 30 minutes, one hour or one day (depending on the situation)? Extra time might change the situation.

Smile – None of this is meant to be confrontational so ask these questions with a smile.

You can ask the health professional to write down what they are saying if it's hard to take it in. Or phone a friend – sometimes just by talking it through out loud, you will decide what to do. Remember you can also ask for five minutes to talk it through alone with your birth partner: by having that space to allow the new situation to sink in and have a hug, it can help acceptance of the new direction of your birth journey or solidify your resolve to continue on your chosen path.

If there is an urgent situation, you need to be able to trust your medical providers to make the right choices. In most cases, there are signals that intervention might be required, but sometimes there is simply not the time to have a measured discussion of risks and benefits. It is possible to feel empowered while also trusting another's decision making, but this is more easily achieved where there is an established relationship with the medical provider. If you have any worries about an aspect of care antenatally, you could ask to speak to a consultant midwife who can co-create a birth plan with you.

The more you are able to educate yourself ahead of time about different scenarios, the less surprises there will be. I acknowledge that there is a fine line between having enough information to feel adequately prepared and feeling overwhelmed by everything that *may*, but probably *won't* happen. It's advisable to read up as much as you can during the second trimester when you can learn at your own pace with no pressure about due dates looming. In the first twelve weeks you may feel that it's too early and perhaps be coping with nausea and fatigue. In the last trimester, it's ideal to switch off from the neocortex and focus on the positive practices of movement, relaxation and mindfulness.

JENNIE'S BIRTHING STORY

(breech, caesarean)

Jennie is a social worker and is a born advocate, but usually for other people! I was impressed with her tenacity in keeping options open for her birth, as it took an expected turn at the end of pregnancy.

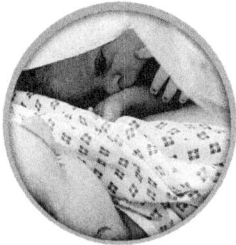

Noah's Birth:

After having made all the arrangements to have a homebirth for our first baby, inevitably our 'plans' went out the window when at 36 weeks we established Noah was in the Frank breech position (folded like a V shape). The homebirth team were no longer able to support me, and the local hospital would only offer me an elective caesarean due to their staff's lack of experience and confidence in delivering breech babies naturally.

I tried everything (spinning babies, moxibustion, acupuncture, External Cephalic Version, visualisation) between 36 weeks and his birth to get Noah to turn but he is clearly stubborn like his mum and lazy like his dad as he didn't budge a centimetre.

Being the dog with a bone that I am, I researched all our options and quickly established there was no reason we could not attempt for a vaginal breech birth (VBB) (it was as safe, Noah was in best position, etc.) except finding the care provider with the right experience to support us. After a three-week battle with NHS trusts, we got the agreement that the John Radcliffe (Oxford) would accept the transfer of our care to their specialist breech team who support VBBs.

I met a couple of their amazing staff for my transfer appointment and clarified our plan, and I strongly suspect that it was after this meeting and knowing things were sorted out that my body relaxed enough for Noah to feel safe enough to make his way.

So, on Saturday, in the early hours of the morning, I began to have 'tightenings' that were like strong period pains. I noticed them but assumed that it was just Braxton Hicks upping their ante. I attended yoga and a baby first aid course that day without any real issue. Then by 9pm Saturday I was getting suspicious as the tightenings were coming regularly (approximately every six minutes for 40 seconds) and were a bit stronger, so I used some breathing techniques at times. I began to time them, and then accepted I was perhaps in early stages of labour (and had been all Saturday).

Sunday morning, I suspected things had died off a bit, as tightenings were more sporadic. However low and behold at 8.30am I felt a pop whilst lying in bed and when I stood up my waters had broken. By 9.30am contractions were every five minutes and stronger so I put my TENS machine on and we set off for Oxford (the midwives didn't want to delay me coming in with him being breech).

When I arrived at the John Radcliffe, contractions were every 2–3 minutes, and I continued to labour for approximately another eight hours. I only ever used the TENS machine and a birth pool for pain relief, and I put this down to the breathing techniques, birth affirmations and education I had learnt and practised during pregnancy both at yoga and antenatal classes.

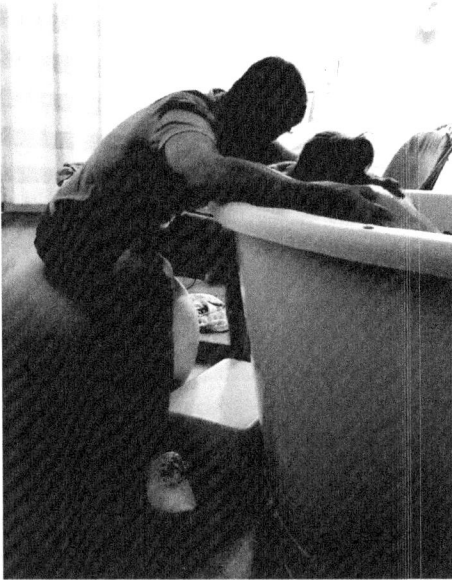

The midwives made comments throughout my labour about how calm and in control I was, just breathing through contractions. I was very quiet and 'in the zone'.

It was funny as at various points in labour I could hear Tessa reminding me to keep breathing, imagine the golden thread/rope/ chain, to keep my jaw loose, and com-menting things like, "I trust my body and my baby to work together", which I really believed. I stayed mostly kneeling or on all fours, as it helped reserve energy but also meant I could do a lot of rocking, swaying and almost 'dancing' with my hips.

I had a really hands-off labour with no examinations or interventions until the very end, when it was confirmed I was 10cm dilated, but despite everyone's best efforts (and all my energy) Noah would just not come down into the birth canal. They could see his buttocks appearing when I contracted but then he would disappear again. After over an hour of my body pushing for him, we all agreed that something was stopping him from coming down and that a c-section was the right option (assisted delivery is not an option with breech babies).

I was lucky to have an amazing consultant and midwives who respected and advocated for all my wishes for a more gentle c-section, so Noah was eventually born at 7.39pm with delayed

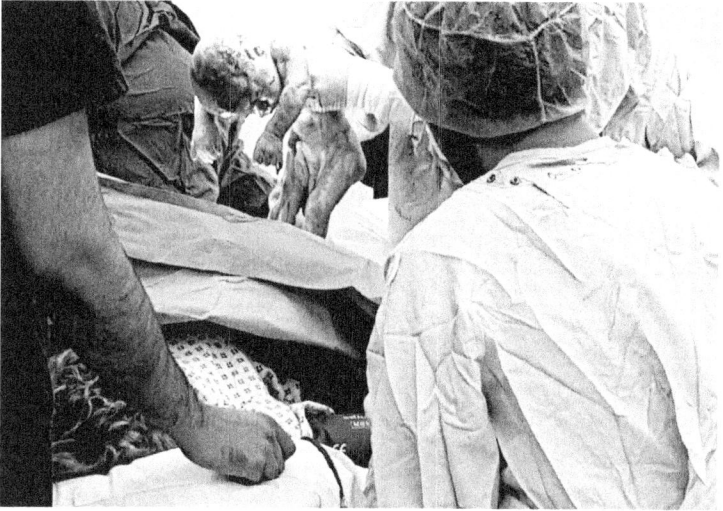

cord clamping, immediate skin-to-skin (where he stayed for the whole op), no cleaning, minimal noise, lowered screen so we saw his sex for ourselves, and not being taken to be weighed until I was all stitched up.

Noah is gorgeous and I have absolutely no regrets about the way his birth ended up. The fight at the end of pregnancy was worth it as the whole labour was an amazing, positive experience and not one to be scared of.

The morals of this birth story that I wanted to share are:

- *do your research.*
- *fight for your wishes as it's your body, your birth and your baby.*
- *accept that there is no 'right' way to birth your baby.*
- *your baby and body know what they are doing, and sometimes it is not aligned with what you may want! However, trust them.*

- *put in serious commitment to learning and practicing breathing techniques if you want to avoid other types of pain relief.*

- *keep breathing, keep calm and keep moving.*

Jennie's birth story is so powerful because although the birth was not the one that she had pictured, her self-advocacy led to a one hundred per cent positive and respectful birthing. She sought out caregivers who were able to support her choices. As women, our way of being is formed, in part, in relation to the masculine. Gender disparity is still very much alive and well. A recent (non-birthing) example is that when my daughter was studying inventors at school aged six, she kept telling me about which ones she'd learnt about that day and every single one of them over a month-long period was male. (Of course, I took in our *Women in Science* book!)

At a young age we can receive the message that innovation, expertise or authority is a male domain, and unless we question these messages, they subconsciously affect how we are in the world. How does this relate to birth? Do we put our trust wholly in medicine-centred practice where birth can be seen as a potential hazard to be managed or in the traditional midwife-led woman-centred care? Perhaps you will find your own balance of the two. My intention is not to say that one is always better than the other, but to say that there is a spectrum of what birth looks like in the UK and worldwide. I encourage you to find your own way through information-gathering and reflection.

In the last chapter, I talked about the 'Mother Wound'. Similarly, there can be a 'Father Wound', where a father was absent, physically or emotionally, or overstepped boundaries in some way, such as being an overbearingly authoritative figure. If there was a deficit in the relationship with your father, you may reflect on how you might project that onto a male birth partner or a male (or female) health professional. Very occasionally I have heard shockingly undermining behaviour used by male consultants, such as the doctor turning to the husband and saying, "Tell your wife to be a good girl." Typing that makes my whole body clench. In the vulnerability of birth, it is much harder to stand up to this sort of dismissive behaviour and to advocate for yourself because you are already dealing with a major physical challenge. If you know that under pressure, you have a tendency to abdicate your voice and sovereignty to someone else, you can prepare your birth partner to back you up and be your voice where needed.

Sometimes we also need to be discerning about our own tendencies. One way of examining these is through shadow archetypes. Carl Jung used this concept to talk about the 'dark side' of our psyches. It refers to that sensation of internal conflict that you may experience when you are frustrated, scared, insecure, or angry. Caroline Myss has written extensively on archetypes and is an easier starting point for exploring how our shadow side may influence decision-making, including around birth. For example, the Prostitute archetype wants acceptance by the tribe and will compromise her values for that. This may show up as "I would love to have a homebirth, but I know my family would be horrified so I won't think about that." If the Child archetype is dominant, you may say "Am I allowed to have a waterbirth?", seeking permission and expecting to have to justify your decision.

You may recognise the shadow archetypes in your birth partners too. The Victim archetype may have a tendency to catastrophise and not want to trouble people with your needs: "If we don't go for the induction now, we might wind the midwives up or they won't be able to fit us in later. Better just to do what they say." One more example: the Saboteur archetype shows up as being sensible and logical, but may stop you trusting your instincts and heart's desire because they want hard evidence for everything: "If you can show me the latest statistics for different birth locations, I might consider it (but it's unlikely)." Archetypes can help us understand patterns of behaviour and enable us to engage more easily with the positive side of our psyches.

📖 REFLECTIONS ⟩ on Discernment

The following reflections are useful in helping you determine your ability to discern what needs to happen in a particular situation. This might be more to do with your ability to get the information or the responsibility of making a decision.

In what situations have you not consented in the past? When has your "No" been overridden with a "Yes" (or "Maybe") by yourself or others? What's stopped your "No" being heard?

How do you react to health professionals? Do you get white coat syndrome (feeling stressed, blood pressure elevating) and how could you manage that during the birthing journey?

How confident do you or your birth partner feel about asking for more information about sweeps, induction, different types of pain relief or any other kind of intervention? How could you feel better prepared to acquire the information you need?

If there is a last-minute change of plan, where would you seek information or support on what your choices are? Who is knowledgeable and can signpost you to the right information or knows what the local policies are in local hospitals? Which websites do you feel have trustworthy information that aligns with your approach to birth?

Journal about the father you needed as a child, the father you need now and may not have. How can you father yourself? (E.g. being clear on your own boundaries to keep you safe.)

There are many archetypes, but did any of those described above resonate with you? If so, how are they showing up in pregnancy? How can you shine a light on that pattern of behaviour and choose to act differently?

SUGGESTIONS

Spend time preparing your birth preferences document and ask your midwife or doula about local policies on issues that concern you.

Print out the BRAINS questions to add to your hospital bag – Go to **www.pearlsofbirthwisdom.com/downloads** for a downloadable PDF.

RESOURCES

www.aims.org.uk is a good place to find information on all aspects of birth.

Watch the 'Consent: It's as Simple as Tea' YouTube video.

Beverley A Lawrence Beech (2014) *Am I Allowed?* AIMS. (Also downloadable as an e-book.)

Rachel Reed (2018) *Why Induction Matters*. Pinter & Martin.

Sheena Byrom and Soo Downe (eds) (2015) *The Roar Behind the Silence: Why Kindness, Compassion and Respect Matter in Maternity Care*. Pinter & Martin.

www.sarawickham.com (Midwife and researcher with excellent articles on many topics, including induction.)

Sue Monk Kidd (2016) *The Dance of the Dissident Daughter: A Woman's Journey from Christian Tradition to the Sacred Feminine*. (A brilliant telling of a woman's questioning of where power comes from.)

Milli Hill (2019) *Give Birth Like a Feminist*. HQ. (I'm not sure that I would personally read this during pregnancy, but it is sadly an accurate description of the service in the UK currently.)

Steve Biddulph (2004) *Manhood: A Guidebook for Men*. Vermillion or (2018) *Raising Boys in the 21ˢᵗ Century*. Thorsons. (I currently cannot find a book I would recommend on the Father Wound, but thoroughly recommend Steve's books about positive masculinity.)

Caroline Myss (2014) *Archetypes: Who are you? A Guide to your Inner-net*. Hay House.

Pearl 7
Time

By nature, we are cyclical beings. Ebb and flow are intrinsic to our human experience.

Imagine a woman's surges have been coming on and off over the last 24 hours. She's been resting as much as she can and balancing her feelings of excitement with patience. The surges have never been coming closer than ten minutes apart and she wonders how long this pre-labour will go on for! The first midwife on the phone wanted her to come in for an induction since she was already overdue, but now the homebirth midwife has arrived and said that there are signs that she is moving into the second stage of labour. The contractions are still ten minutes apart. Half an hour later her baby boy is born.

In the hospital notes, there is guidance about when to ring the triage line that makes it sound as if every labour will follow a set pattern: the contractions will be so many minutes apart and lasting so many seconds. This makes most people unsurprisingly obsessed with timing the contractions so that they get permission to travel into hospital and has given rise to apps that record your surges. As Hester found in a previous birth story, focusing on timing can prove to be a great distraction and make it harder to cope with the contractions. The truth is that the pattern of contractions can vary from individual to individual and they do not predict how long it will be before you meet your baby.

For many women, hospital policies determine what happens during pregnancy and birth. Around the world, what is considered the due date varies. A fixed date, rather than a range of normality, can cause a lot of negative feelings and a push towards induction. Policies will also vary across hospitals, for example how long overdue a baby can be and still have a homebirth, or when an induction is booked for. These policies are based on normal practice and not always good research. A policy is a written document that outlines the exact requirements in a given situation. It is a route of practice a midwife must take, *unless* the mother requests otherwise. For example, a woman may have been charting her cycle prior to pregnancy and knows within a few days of when conception happened. She may find that this does not match her due date and therefore is happy to decline induction and go beyond the estimated due date; waiting for her baby/body to initiate the labour. Perhaps women could be given a due week or fortnight to provide a wider window of when to expect labour to start to avoid the feeling of pressure mounting if the due date comes and goes with no sign of labour starting.

Everything is timed and monitored: the contractions, when the contractions started, how dilated the cervix is, the temperature of the birth pool, the length of pushing, how long before the cord was cut, the length of time between the baby being born and the placenta arriving...just writing this makes me feel slightly stressed! Hopefully this is all going on without the mother's notice, but it has an impact. The body senses a lack of safety when there are time pressures, and this may prevent dilation from occurring or even the baby moving down. I wonder if many instrumental births could be avoided if physical and psychological safety was paramount: not in the sense of clinical indication and birth statistics, but a respect for the biological process at work and a minimum of disturbance to it.

Here are two birth stories about timing, including a positive induction.

RUTH'S BIRTHING STORY

(long first phase)

Ruth is a teacher and an open-minded person, whom I really enjoyed having in my classes. This is the birth story, via Facebook messenger, of her second daughter.

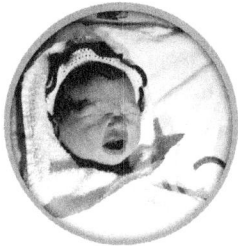

Cally's Birth:

4ᵗʰ May 10.18am

Ruth: Hi Tessa, my waters broke last night, but no contractions! I've got until ten tonight before an induction that I'd really rather avoid! I'm bouncing on my birth ball, and kept my daughter out of nursery so I can breastfeed her as much as possible, and I've got some jasmine oil in a diffuser – any other tips for kick-starting contractions?! xx

Tessa: Look at the Spinning Babies website and the forward inversion technique. Do you think it's because baby's not engaging? I would also try the side lying release and standing release on the same website. Also, in case baby's finding it difficult to get over pelvic brim, start from cat, go into forearms and 'walk' the knees as far back as you can without collapsing. This can also be done in the bath/birth pool. Thinking of you xx

Ruth: *Baby feels like she engages for a bit then moves out again (based on pressure in my pelvis). The inversion felt like it helped, will give the others a try too. Thank you! xx*

4*th* May 3.22pm

Ruth: *Having some contractions now, though not all that regular yet - the side lying release seemed really helpful, then did about an hour of dancing which started contractions off! They were stopping when I stopped dancing, but had a few now while I'm just sat down so starting to feel positive xx*

Tessa: *Is there anything you feel hasn't been sorted out? Do you feel your daughter is looked after in the way YOU need? Can you ask your baby if there's anything she needs from you to get started? Trust your inner voice. Sending so much positivity xx*

Ruth: *Honestly feeling like everything is good, think sleep might actually be the missing factor, might try a nap. Thank you so much xx*

5*th* May 9.22am

Ruth: *Hi Tessa, turns out my body knew what was needed more than I did. I thought we would have a lovely straight forward delivery, just like we did with the first and that this could all happen at home. In fact, this baby was nearly 9lbs and contained in a huge amount of amniotic fluid that for the most part, wasn't breaking.*

After a small water leak on Wednesday night, I spent Thursday trying to get baby to engage, lots of our poses were really useful, but the main thing that worked was dancing! Even after all of that though, nothing was consistent. The amazing home-birth team came out Thursday evening and were fantastic.

Having examined me, they realised there was unbroken water between baby and my cervix so she wasn't able to engage. If nothing happened spontaneously, I'd need these waters broken. We held off as long as we could, but had to accept that this would happen. Before leaving home, I played briefly in the birth pool with my daughter, partly because she'd been so excited about it, partly so I could come to terms with not having my ideal birth.

Despite being in the delivery suite (as we were more than 24 hours since waters had broken) our midwife was lovely, respected my wishes and acted as a shield between ourselves and the very medical doctor! After my waters were broken (massively flooding the floor!!) contractions started but still not very regular.

There was talk of hormonal induction, which I very much wanted to avoid, but baby's heart rate was dropping and ultimately we were going to do whatever was best for her. I breathed my way through contractions using all of our visualisation techniques, particularly that of the opening flower.

Then believe it or not, the moment our midwife had to call the doctor in to authorise the drip, I felt the urge to push. Baby Cally was out shortly after afterwards with the help of the golden rope/chain breath and the waves on the beach visualisation.

There was no way could I have done this birth at home with my toddler "helping" and I'm so grateful for my body knowing this and resisting my desires to push it into established labour. I'm also, as ever, grateful for the visualisation techniques you've taught us and which helped me through the strongest contractions with just gas and air when needed.

Thank you! Honestly wouldn't have done it without you – again! Also meant to say no stiches this time despite baby being huge! Definitely put this down to yoga.

xx

Ruth's birthing story shows how labour doesn't always fit a neat template. The birth of her first child also showed this: Ruth was booked into my birth preparation workshop on a Saturday afternoon, but texted to say she was having contractions on the Thursday before and so would unfortunately miss it. Imagine my surprise when she walked into the room still very much pregnant on the Saturday! Ruth said that her contractions had been coming regularly and they'd travelled into the hospital, but when she got there, she didn't like it and the contractions faded. They were sent back home to wait for things to pick up again. I'm pleased to say that after the workshop, Ruth's surges re-started, and her first baby girl was born later that night.

KATIA'S BIRTHING STORY

(induction)

Katia is a yoga teacher and loves being active, whether it's teaching spinning, cycling around town or taking the dog for a walk. She is a natural people-person and made firm friends in the pregnancy yoga class with other expectant mums.

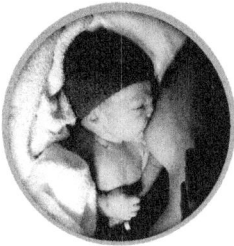

Noah's Birth:

I was due to be induced on 26th October at 40 weeks. The reason was that I was over 40 at the time of conception and so current medical advice is to not go over the due date. I'd had no other complications during pregnancy (if you don't count hyperemesis which they don't in relation to labour) and I'm pretty sure this advice will change in the future but it's where we are now.

I spoke to a number of people including the various midwives who supported me through the pregnancy, fellow yoga teachers with pregnancy experience, friends and family about the pros and cons of induction. It was useful to know that I didn't have to do it. It was a choice and I could change my mind right up to the day if I didn't want to be induced – as long as the baby was happy and safe of course.

On my 39th week I opted to have two sweeps to see if they could get labour started. I experienced some cramps after both sweeps but neither turned into labour. I was pretty uncomfortable by this time so was using as many techniques as possible, both proved and unproved, to bring on labour including daily dog walks up hill, climbing stairs, squats, eating pineapple and curries, sniffing and massaging clary sage and bouncing on my Pilates ball! I really was quite ready for this baby to arrive – not least because I was still suffering with the nausea of the first trimester, which never really left me; this was the biggest pregnancy challenge for me without a doubt.

Saturday 26th arrived and the hospital rang me promptly at 9.30am to book me in for induction at 3pm that same day. Nathan, my partner, drove us in to RBH with just a small bag of provisions for our appointment. On the ward they carried out a couple of checks on me and monitored baby's heart rate for 20 minutes or so. This was the first stage of induction which is administered by pessary, which is like a tampon and sits next to the mouth of your cervix, and releases hormones (prostaglandins) to stimulate labour. There were a couple of things that I didn't know at this stage including:

- *When inserting the pessary, the midwife can break your waters for you – this would further guarantee the imminent arrival of your baby but rule out the possibility of going home.*

- *Having the induction ruled me out for going into the midwife-led unit – this is because the likelihood of needing other interventions increases (I knew the second part of this but not the first bit as I'd assumed I could still start on the midwife-led unit).*

- *We should have taken our labour bags with us as they could've insisted that I stayed in hospital from this point onwards – we hadn't realised this so most upsettingly for Nathan had left the painstakingly-prepared snack bag at home!*

I'd insisted to the midwife that I wanted to go home after the pessary was fitted – mainly because I really wanted a jacket potato and as they can take 10 – 24 hours to work I'd seen that this was usually an option. She was a little unsure but after checking with the consultant they said yes we could go home, so after a short walk around the hospital to check I didn't have any adverse effects we got back in the car and went home in time for Strictly Come Dancing and the tuna jacket potato that I was so craving.

After managing half my dinner and not quite seeing the end of "Strictly" [Come Dancing], my cramps had ramped up into pretty strong contractions. It seemed a bit unbelievable that it could happen so fast, and so, Nathan rang the hospital to see what they said. As I was in a fair amount of discomfort, we went in to be assessed. This was quite a challenging process as in order to monitor the baby, they wanted me to lie on a bed for 20 minutes or so, which I just couldn't do. I just wanted to move around in the way we'd practised in the pregnancy yoga classes and try to breathe as much as possible. I felt very hot and irritable at this stage, but having got some measurements, they confirmed that I was 2cms dilated and so sent me down to the Marsh ward in order for labour to progress.

Supporting me to the lift, the midwife and Nathan walked me down to Marsh ward – all the while I was having contractions and making small puddles around the hospital for which I was apologising profusely for. There was another, very friendly, midwife called Christina. I was led into a room and the two midwives were discussing my handover when suddenly my waters broke and the noise I was making during contractions apparently changed to a more 'pushing' sound. Christina reassessed me and announced me to be 6cms dilated and promptly waved me off to the delivery suite.

I remember having an internal dialogue of 'no, no, no I don't want to be in labour and I don't want this baby to come – it's all a terrible idea – what was I thinking? This then passed as I became focused on the pushing and the process again supported by the midwives. In my third room for the day, two midwives supported me through the second phase of labour, which is the actual pushing stage. I actually preferred this stage as each push felt like a bit of relief as it was accompanied by more amniotic fluid and a step closer to meeting this baby. I used as many upright positions as I could remember from Tessa's classes plus a couple suggested by the midwives. I was squeezing Nathan's hand throughout and very focused as it's such an all-consuming process. It was very intense but at any points where I felt I couldn't do it, Nathan and the midwives encouraged me on, and baby Arlo made an appearance an hour and a half later at 1.06am. 7lb 6oz.

I was shell shocked by the whole thing and how quick it had been, and my body was shaking for a good hour, from all the adrenaline, working hard to process everything for me. I have to be honest and say we didn't get to use all the techniques we'd learned and didn't even open the snack bag (!) But my body did adapt to the demands placed upon it and my mind came around a few hours later. Induction was a positive experience for me.

Induction sometimes get a negative press in natural birth circles. However, like Katia's, I do hear positive stories of labours that have been induced for a range of reasons. I like how she's shared what she learnt about induction retrospectively for the benefit of other expectant mums and suggest that you ask for a comprehensive explanation of the possible consequences of going down that route. Unless you've been induced before with synthetic oxytocin, you can't be sure how strongly your body will respond to it and how far away you were from a natural start to labour (my impression from hearing hundreds of birth stories is that those who felt closer to the baby being ready to be born found induction less challenging because their body was already gearing up for labour).

By the start of the twentieth century, it was commonplace in Western culture to think about the body as a machine. This was helpful to some degree because it encouraged detailed study of the body's mechanisms, but it is unhelpful inasmuch as we expect the body to behave in standard ways. I commonly observe in the birth preparation workshops that partners expect the labour to start, they will quickly transfer to the hospital and the midwife will handle everything. However, the majority of labours start at home and the birth partner will usually be the sole support until the contractions are closer together, which may take some time. If this person has some basic understanding of physiological birth and how it is as much a psychological process as a physical one, they can set the scene for the rest of birthing journey by supporting the individual, rather than a 'machine' that's expected to 'work' a certain way and in specific time frames.

As the contractions start, it is really important to not get too excited, too soon. They may be regular and already feeling quite intense, but you'll know when you've shifted into active labour because you won't be able to think about anything else and will need to give all your focus to them. In that first phase, try to potter as normal until you need to give your focus over to them. If you feel better being still, create a nest of lots of pillows cushioning your head, back, bump and between the legs and have two hot-water bottles: one for where you are feeling the surges most around your bump and one for the lower back. Try to drift off between contractions and rest as much as you can to conserve energy for later. I call this the 'Rest and Nest' phase.

Often women can be frightened of the contractions prior to the labour starting. It can be helpful to remember the ebb and flow analogy: after each contraction, there is an expansion phase where the uterus is at rest. In class we practice mindfulness so that we can stay in the present moment, and during the birthing journey we can focus on this one surge right now, rather than thinking about how many are to come or whether they become more intense. By using the breathing techniques and visualisations (see Box 13 for one), we avoid panicking and are better able to manage the intensity. Contrary to what many people think, rather than avoiding the sensation, we are leaning into it. The techniques help us to relax the body so that tension does not add to what is being felt and the contractions can be effective in bringing our baby into the world.

Contractions, these wonderful surges of physical energy, do not always follow the textbook pattern. I have heard of women whose contractions never get closer than ten minutes apart, right up to the birth of their babies. A wonderful doula local to me, Callie Fontain, told me about another pattern: "I had a first-time mum who had double contractions one immediately after the other, then a long pause in between for around four hours until fully dilated, then she had a resting stage [transition] for at least 20 minutes. When her contractions started again, she had exactly the same rhythm of contractions and worked so hard to utilise each one until her baby was born". She was 1 in 100 of birthing women, but it shows that we are not standardised machines, but individuals with individual bodies that birth differently.

BOX 13: Waves visualisation

Find a comfortable position and relax. Connect with your baby by thinking of your baby in the ideal position for them starting labour: head down, bottom up, chin tucked in. Picture how the proteins in the baby's lungs will activate labour, starting a cascade of hormones to circulate through your body. You feel the first contractions starting: perhaps a tightening, squeezing or pressure around your bump. You also imagine the expansion as the contraction ends and how you can rest.

As you imagine the next surge, visualise it or feel it as a wave washing up your legs towards your pelvis. Picture a powerful ocean wave. At the peak of the surge you can imagine the peak of a wave, and then imagine the water running back down the beach as you rest into the expansion.

You can even picture your womb as a cave and imagine the wave drawing your baby gently but surely down and out into the sunshine. You can feel that the powerful ocean wave is a helpful force of nature and go with it, concentrating on one wave at a time. As the wave recedes you imagine yourself floating, totally relaxed and making the most of the chance to rest, drink some water, say something, change position, whatever supports you.

As you practice this visualisation, you might breathe in as the surge washes up the legs and breathe out as it washes down. During the real birthing journey, you may need to breathe in and out several times during a contraction. When you finish the visualisation, do several pelvic floor squeezes to psychologically seal everything up and picture your baby smiling in your womb, safely tucked under your heart.

I used the Waves visualisation described during the birth of my second child. I was in the bath at home waiting for the pool to be filled downstairs. It wonderfully concentrated my mind. I only discovered the next day that I had been pushing my forehead against the wall strongly enough to have a tender patch. I was totally not aware of the strength of the sensation that made me do that at the time because of the endorphins, the natural pain killers, circulating.

When I hear that someone has had an induction and no artificial pain killers I am in awe. The artificial hormones that are given intravenously or as a pessary do not travel across into the brain unlike the natural ones, so the surges can be more intense, more quickly. However, I have noticed that the experience of induction can vary hugely depending on when in the pregnancy it has been started. If induction has been started before the baby's estimated due date due to medical reasons, it can be harder because the mother's body may not have started preparing for the birth ahead. However, if the baby is 'overdue,' often the mother's body has started preparing and already softening, and her cervix may be partly dilated before the induction starts. Just as physiological births can vary incredibly, so can inductions, so please approach them like anything else, one moment, one breath, one surge at a time.

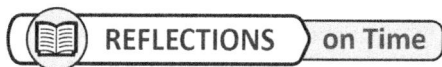

📖 REFLECTIONS ⟩ on Time

These reflections are about understanding how time has affected our approach to birth as a culture and from a medical perspective. You may want to consider your broader relationship to time.

How do you cope with uncertainty? Do you prefer to know exactly when things will happen or are you able to allow things to unfold? What could help you cope with the unknown? (E.g. breathing techniques to soothe the nervous system.)

How do you view the body? As a machine that can be broken and needs to be fixed or regulated? Or as an intelligent mind-body system? How do you think this will affect your approach to the birthing journey?

Has your birth partner become informed enough to support a physiological birth while still at home? How can you both increase your knowledge?

SUGGESTIONS

Search for natural birth or hypnobirth on YouTube to counter all the dramatic ones you've watched on TV over the years. My online birth preparation course contains three diverse ones.

Visit my YouTube Channel Yoga with Tessa at https://www.youtube.com/user/tessavenuti/ and type 'Pregnancy' into the search function to see all the relevant videos including visualisations, yoga sequences and breathing techniques.

Join my mailing list (at www.pearlsofbirthwisdom.com) for Birth Partner's checklist (9 page PDF) on different ways to support you.

RESOURCES

Becky Reed (2016) *Birth in Focus*. Pinter & Martin. (Stories of diverse births and graphic photos of birth that can help prepare you for the visceral nature of labour.)

John O'Donohue (2007) *Benedictus: A Book of Blessings*. Bantam

Press. (This book of poetry is beautiful and contains ones for new mothers and fathers, and for the arrival of a baby, and is a wonderful way to spend time as you await the birth).

www.sarawickham.com (Search for 'fixed point due date' for information on the benefits of a wider window around due dates).

Articles on how the body is constructed as a machine in medicine and Western society in general:

https://undark.org/2016/07/06/mind-machine-medicine-militaristic-healthcare/

https://evmed.asu.edu/blog/body-not-machine

Pearl 8
Stillness

By stopping and becoming still, a deep listening is possible. Undistracted by thoughts you sense what the body needs.

Imagine that through your reflections and preparation you have reached a place of stillness within yourself: the stillness that comes from knowing that you have done all that you can, and the rest is providence. You have gathered those around you that can give you the support you need and, whilst going in the unknown, the desire to see this child gives you the confidence that you are headed in the right direction.

Today as I was teaching in class, the wind was rattling the external doors and blowing autumnal leaves around. All the women were lying down for relaxation and were so still and settled. There was such a juxtaposition with what was happening outside that I incorporated it into the yoga nidra (relaxation) I was delivering. Experiencing the movement of wind as we breathed in and the stillness inside as we breathed out.

We can be at peace with the unknown, the discomfort, the changing situation. How would it feel to simultaneously experience movement and stillness, just as there might be in different parts of the birthing? Like your emotions changing hour by hour as you wait for labour to start, but a deeper confidence and knowledge that the surges will start when the time is right. Or maybe the health professionals moving around preparing the space and at the same time you are deeply focused, one-pointed, on the breath to manage the waves of intensity. Or like the midwife managing the birth of the placenta while you gaze transfixed at your newborn, oblivious to what's going on around you.

A formal meditation practice teaches people to observe what is happening without judgement or reaction, whether it is thoughts that constantly pop up in the mind, sensations wanting our attention in the body, or external stimuli distracting us. However, it's not necessary to have years of this formal seated meditation practice to benefit from mindfulness. In the pregnancy yoga classes we develop mindfulness through paying attention to the breath and how the body feels in the postures and movements that we do.

Although as a teacher I am observing to see that someone doesn't put themselves in danger by overloading a joint, doing something that will aggravate an old injury or exacerbate their blood pressure issue for example, I hand the responsibility to the woman to determine what feels comfortable and pleasing to do on that day. If her energy is lower, she might come out of a posture sooner. Or if the baby is in a position that makes a movement uncomfortable, the mother lets me know so that I can adapt what we are doing to make her comfortable.

By developing a deep listening to our bodies, we are able to relax into the knowledge that we will very likely know what helps us to be as comfortable as possible during the birth journey. When someone knows their body intimately through this mindfulness, she is more likely to trust her intuition about what will support her body and she will take ownership over what is happening in her journey through this rite of passage.

Here is the story of the births of three daughters, by both parents.

SARAH'S BIRTHING STORIES

(one hospital, two homebirths)

Sarah is one of those people that you'd call first in a crisis. As a scientist she likes to have as much information at her fingertips as possible before making a decision.

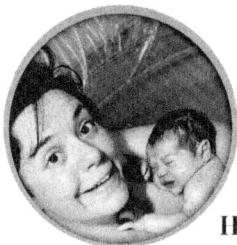

Harriet (Hattie)'s birth:

My first pregnancy went very smoothly all the way through, and when thinking about where and how I would give birth I was keen to aim for as natural a birth as possible, but while also trying to be realistic as to what might happen. I was slightly daunted by the unknown, but also found that I felt fairly confident leading up to the birth that my body knew what to do.

I went to pregnancy yoga classes and learnt about the importance of breathing and relaxation, I read a few pregnancy and birth books and was particularly encouraged by reading Ina May Gaskin talk about her experiences as a midwife, and the conditions conducive to a natural birth. As a biologist, the interplay between adrenaline and oxytocin was fascinating to me, the way these two different hormones work against each other and how you stimulate one and avoid the other, appealed to both my scientific logical mind and also my pregnant self! For each of my labours I held on to the belief that wherever I was, if I felt safe and secure, this would give me the best chance of a smooth delivery.

I was nine days past my 'due date' when I started to feel aches in my back that morning, which gradually progressed to something more rhythmic. After lunch we went for a walk, and somehow the afternoon passed with some bouncing on the birth ball, watching TV and at some point, I tried out the TENS machine. The plan was to stay at home as long as I could, before heading into the hospital and hopefully to the midwife-led unit for a more 'home-like' environment. After calling the hospital and being told to come in (when the contractions reached a certain frequency), Chris made sure we both ate dinner (which was very wise – I could easily have not bothered but as it turned out we needed the energy as we would be up all night!).

Later that evening we went into hospital but were sent home again as I wasn't "far along enough". Of course, as soon as we got home again things started to get more intense and it wasn't long before we were back again and "allowed" to stay this time – by now it was the early hours of the morning. The difficulty of going to and from the hospital would become one of the reasons why we were both so keen on the idea of homebirth in subsequent pregnancies – not least because those car journeys were some of the most uncomfortable I've ever experienced!

Once the midwives established that my labour had progressed far enough, they discussed our options, and having read the birth plan we'd written, they already had a good idea what my preferences were and had been working out how to help me with them even before we got to the discussion. This made me so glad we'd written the plan. Even though we heard lots about how no labour ever goes to plan, I wanted to make sure everything was explained so that I didn't have to try and put it into words at the time! And it more than did its job. The birth plan said that I really wanted to use a birthing pool, but the pools on the unit were in use. By the time we were told this, they had already come up with an alternative, which was an inflatable pool in the delivery suite, which I was really grateful for.

Rayanne, the midwife looking after us, said she was so pleased to be able to help with a straightforward water birth, as most of those she attended on the delivery suite were more complicated. The room was a bit cramped with the pool in there along with the bed and everything else, but it was calm, private and quiet, and for the next few hours as I laboured, there was Chris holding my hand, and Rayanne who took a fantastically hands-off approach, mainly just observing and commenting/reassuring me when needed. She listened to the baby's heartbeat every so often and that was it.

The gas and air really helped: partly I really enjoyed the slightly dreamy state it produced, and partly it was probably something to do to keep the rhythm in my breathing and focus attention on! Chris held my hand, offered me water (and the occasional piece of Kendal mint cake, which was amazing for a sugar hit without having to really eat, which I didn't want to do), and kept me calm and focused. I have no idea how long this part of labour lasted, the gas and air and the labour haze made it all a bit fuzzy!

I felt things change when my waters burst, the weight of the baby was suddenly lower, and pressing harder against my pelvis. I didn't know that's what had happened, but I remember hearing Rayanne saying to Chris, "That was the waters going" and she said to me, "That feels different now doesn't it?" and I remember thinking, not for the last time, how does she know that's how I'm feeling?

The amazing thing about the midwives that supported me in each labour was that they seemed to be able to tell what was going on without any physical examinations or measurements, they could just tell, from the way I responded to contractions or *what I was saying. They used their experience and their knowledge to judge what stage labour was at, and what was likely to happen next, which allowed them to leave me to labour without intervention, and also, thinking back, probably helped me feel much more relaxed and confident, because of how confident they were.*

The pushing stage took quite a bit longer the first time (I also remember Rayanne saying, part way through, next time it will be much easier! I wasn't really sure I wanted to think about that then!!). The baby's head kept coming out and then sinking back in between contractions, and at one point I remember her saying something like; "We'll give it a bit longer and if you've not made some more progress we'll need to get you out of the pool and examine you.". I have no idea whether she was intentionally trying to give me a push (!) to find some last reserves of energy, but either way it worked!

I was determined this baby was going to be born in the pool, so with those last few contractions I held on, and at last there she was! The most incredible feeling each time was that sudden change from the most intense effort and pain (I'm not going to pretend it was just uncomfortable – it hurt!) I've ever experienced, to the feeling of this baby slipping out of me and the euphoria of them coming up to meet me out of the water! We have some amazing photos of that moment, where I held my daughter for the first time.

Afterwards Chris cut the cord, we got out of the pool, lay on the bed and got wrapped up in lots of towels and blankets, I tried to feed but she wasn't having any of it – still a bit too sleepy! It took me a while to deliver the placenta. In the end Rayanne realised it was because I hadn't been to the toilet for a long time and my full bladder was stopping it coming out. Once that was sorted it came away easily – another one of those midwife instinct moments, which saved all kinds of further complications! I had a few stitches while Chris held the baby and phoned the proud grandparents. Then I had a shower and we were taken up to the postnatal ward with our new daughter.

Hattie was born at 4.58am, and as everything had been straightforward, I was hopeful that I would be able to go home later that day. However, she didn't take to breastfeeding quickly, and while she would latch on she wasn't actually sucking much at all, so I was told we had to stay in "until feeding was established". I envied the mum in the next bed who had had her second baby who was feeding fine and went home after a few hours although I was trapped in the overheated maternity ward while Chris went home.

After a full day and a night in which neither me nor Hattie had got much sleep, and I'd been told I should start to express some milk for her, I decided I was going home, where we had a pump, and where Chris would be able to hold her while I used it! This was another part of the decision to plan a homebirth the second time around, so that we could be in the comfort of our own home where, thanks to those hormones again, I would be more able to establish breastfeeding when I didn't feel like I was being examined all the time.

Martha's birth:

When I was pregnant again 18 months later, Chris and I knew almost without discussing it that we would be planning a homebirth. I joined the local homebirth support group, found out how to borrow a birth pool, and from the first booking appointment

I said I wanted to have the baby at home. Everyone was very supportive (second time mum, straightforward first labour and so on), until the midwife noticed from my notes that I had lost a lot of blood the first time, primarily because of how long it took to deliver the placenta. There were clear reasons for this which could be avoided this time, but it still took some discussion and conversations with the consultant midwife before we could be given the go ahead to have the baby at home.

The other potential problem was that there was no dedicated homebirth team at the time (which there is now), and so it was potluck when you went into labour as to whether there would be a suitably experienced midwife able to attend. If there was no one, then you had to come into the hospital after all. This uncertainty definitely doesn't help with the oxytocin levels! Anyway, we went ahead, made plans for Hattie to be looked after, borrowed towels, bought shower curtains, wrote a birth plan, made a playlist, and waited.

My due date was six days before Hattie's birthday, I wasn't expecting the baby to be on time but was hoping there would at least be a bit of a gap between their birthdays! However, the baby had other plans – on Hattie's birthday, 10ᵗʰ March, at six days overdue, I saw the midwife who found I was already 2cm dilated, which was quite a surprise as I hadn't felt anything at all yet! She did a stretch and sweep as well and sent me off to see what happened. After a few aches and tightenings Thursday night, we went to bed as normal, but Chris decided it would be wise to work from home the next day rather than going into London!

At about 7.30 the following morning, sitting in bed with Hattie, I started to feel the aching coming back, and although very mild and not with any pattern to it, I began to feel this was it and made sure Chris stuck to his decision to work from home. After breakfast I left Chris working and took Hattie off to the park. A 30-minute walk there and back (as well as a bit of lifting a toddler on and off swings!) helped things progress, and by the time we got back two hours later, the contractions were coming about every 5–7 minutes.

Chris had inflated the birth pool while we were out, we had lunch, put Hattie down for her nap, and I rang the RBH to let them know and check if a midwife was available to come out to us at home. I was told they would contact the community midwifes and get back to us. Meanwhile we got the TENS machine out, I bounced on my birth ball and we called my parents to tell them to come and get Hattie, who was completely refusing to nap and was chatting away to her toys upstairs!

About an hour after I first called the hospital, contractions were closer together and getting stronger all the time, but we still hadn't had a call back, so Chris rang again to tell them things were progressing and find out what the situation for homebirth was. We were told someone could come out and assess me when we needed it but warned that the overnight shift didn't have enough experienced midwives so there wasn't anyone to attend a homebirth after 7.30pm that night, and that Rushey, the midwife-led unit, would also be closed. This was disappointing, but we were starting to think it wouldn't be a problem given how quickly things seemed to be going! We were told to ring back at the point we would have gone into hospital, and they would get someone to come out to do an assessment.

Chris set about filling the pool, which involved a lot of boiling water in pans on the hob as we only have a water tank which needed time to re-fill. It felt a little like a scene from "Call the Midwife"! My parents came to collect Hattie about 2.30, and by then contractions were getting quite intense and it was taking all my concentration to breathe through them. I took some paracetamol and turned the TENS up, and Chris rang the hospital again and asked them to send a midwife to come and assess how things were going.

We were conscious all this time that we didn't want to have to transfer to hospital at the last minute if things were still going by 7.30, and I knew I would cope a lot better with having to go in if I was prepared for it happening. Perhaps the rate things progressed was down to me subconsciously trying to avoid going anywhere, who knows.

The lovely Julie arrived about 3.15pm having been called away from her antenatal clinic down the road, and on examining me found I was 4cm dilated. "You're definitely in labour", she said, although I have to admit I was a little disappointed not to be further along by this point, given the intensity of the contractions! I got into the pool about 3.30pm. After some phone calls, Julie confirmed that she would now stay with us to deliver our baby, and that her colleague would join us when their clinic was finished just after 5pm, to be here for the delivery. She also arranged for someone to come from the hospital with the all-important Entonox! I was preparing myself for another few hours of sitting in the pool, to get through the remaining 6cm.

However, baby had other plans! While Julie sat down at the kitchen table, starting to write up some notes, I'd been in the pool perhaps ten minutes when the sensations changed. I recognised this from my first labour – everything was telling me to push! Despite coping well so far, I freaked out a bit at this point, having just been told I was only 4cm, I was suddenly terrified that I was feeling this urge too soon, but Julie reassured me that if I was ready to push then I should listen to my body and go with it.

I had been telling myself through pregnancy that when this point came I wouldn't let it scare me as it had a bit the first time, as I'd know what was happening, but it came on so suddenly I didn't feel very prepared. This was another of those times where the skill and experience of the midwife really made a difference – even with me progressing from 4cm to pushing that quickly, Julie didn't miss a beat when she said sometimes

167

that's how it happens. There was no need to examine me or ask more questions, she clearly just knew, and trusted my body maybe more than I did at that point!

I remember being in the pool, leaning on the edge as I had with Hattie, with Chris kneeling at the side (this time with some cushions for his knees!), while Chris assured me that the gas and air was definitely on the way. What I didn't know was that Julie was telling him from behind me that there was no chance it would be here before the baby! I'm very glad they were able to communicate that without my knowledge!

We then had a bit of a drama trying to source a hand mirror for Julie to watch the baby crowning – she didn't have her full birth kit with her so we were somewhat making do! After sending Julie searching through our kitchen cupboards, Chris witnessed our daughter's head being born in a small hand-painted decorative mirror which happened to be on a shelf near the pool!!

So, on the strength of two paracetamol and after an active labour of 40 minutes, Martha was born at 4.10pm! She was a little grey and quiet so our skin-to-skin time was a little shorter than intended, then Chris cut the cord and helped me out while Julie got Martha warmed up and checked her over. In hindsight we're very lucky she arrived so smoothly and without any complications, given Julie had no assistance and very little equipment to speak of! About 20 minutes later, a care assistant arrived from the RBH with the birth kit and the gas and air, and sometime after 5pm the second midwife turned up, and Chris answered the door holding the baby!

I was concerned to get the placenta delivered as this took a little too long last time, so I tried to get Martha feeding and she latched on instantly like a pro and fed for a good 20 minutes. It still took quite a while to get the placenta out though, and between this and some stitches, I was definitely thankful that the gas and air had made it at last! I was stitched up sitting on the edge of the sofa with a foot on each of Hattie's small IKEA chairs, by the light of one of our own head torches! For us this kind of characterised the whole homebirth experience – the combination of the more relaxed atmosphere of being in our own environment, with the slightly make-do approach of using whatever came to hand.

Martha was weighed on the kitchen worktop, and the placenta delivered into our washing up bowl! And the midwives then sat for a while writing up their notes at our kitchen table, while Chris emptied and deflated the pool and packed it all away. At some point Julie came across my birth plan, tucked into my maternity notes, and we realised that she'd not even had chance to ask for it, never mind read it.

After that there was nothing else left for the midwives to do but gather up all their equipment, have a last cuddle with the new arrival and head off home for their dinner. By 7.30pm, around 12 hours after the first twinges, we were set in our own home, with everything just as it had been that morning, only now we had a brand-new baby girl in our arms.

Nothing will ever beat that surreal and wonderful feeling of sitting there, thinking about how much had just happened in that room and how much had changed, and yet feeling so completely normal like everything was just as it should be, in our house with our baby. That feeling alone would have made the whole thing worthwhile. We put pizzas in the oven for dinner, made some phone calls, and sent some emails and photos to friends and family, and then went to bed with our little girl.

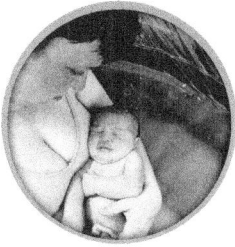

Isabel's birth:

Two and a half years later I was pregnant with our third child, and there was no doubt we wanted to have the baby at home just like Martha. The big change this time was that Reading now had a dedicated homebirth team of experienced midwives supporting women to birth their babies at home. So, we were hopeful that at least some of the obstacles to a homebirth last time around had been removed. The homebirth team were fantastic all the way through, from my first booking appointment, which I had at home while Chris looked after the older two in the other room, right through to the birth itself.

At around 28 weeks pregnant my bump was measuring larger than normal and so began a series of growth scans and tests to make sure nothing was wrong. Happily no problems were found with either me or the baby: no infections and baby was growing nicely. The issue was they were growing a bit too well: on one scan they were off the scale on the centile chart, and I also had developed a condition called polyhydramnios (essentially too much amniotic fluid, often associated with larger babies). These factors together raised questions about our homebirth plans: even once any kind of infection or other cause had mainly been ruled out, the extra fluids meant that the risk of cord prolapse (the umbilical cord coming out before the baby and then becoming trapped by the head and cutting off oxygen supply) was increased. And there were concerns that a larger baby could become stuck during birth. We were advised by a consultant at the hospital that we should have the baby in hospital in the delivery suite. But we knew there was more to it than this.

We knew that while the relative risk of cord prolapse might have doubled, in absolute terms the risk itself was extremely low, especially if the waters didn't go prior to the head engaging, which they hadn't done before. And if they did, we could still go into hospital if we chose to. We also knew that the water levels were likely to go down towards the end of the pregnancy, which in the end they did, and by the time I reached my due date they were back to 'average', so this issue was removed anyway.

The remaining problem was the size of the baby, which is commonly thought to increase the risk of shoulder dystocia (shoulder getting stuck), although the registrar himself admitted that around half of cases of this happen in smaller babies, so there isn't really a clear correlation. We had a long conversation with our named midwife, Dani, about the risks involved in this and what we could do about them. While not contradicting the advice of the consultant, she also talked us through the procedures for releasing the baby if this did happen, and that these could still be done at home if need be.

She also reassured us that many cases of shoulders getting stuck did happen in smaller babies: it isn't so much to do with size as which way the baby starts to come out, which you can control to an extent with active birth and positioning, both beforehand and if there is a problem. I had some ideas already of how I could help with this myself, and we both felt confident in Dani's advice, so were content to go ahead.

The week before and after my due date, I'd been hoping to have a sweep to try and encourage things along. Given how large this baby was I was definitely ready for them to arrive! But we'd never been able to manage it, the head was never engaged so we just had to wait for things to get going on their own. On Tuesday 26th February at just over 41 weeks I tried some nip-

ple stimulation in the morning using my breast pump, and then went for a walk around a nearby National Trust property, just as I did before my first daughter was born, and did a lot of long strides and squats (luckily the gardens weren't too busy!!). The combination of this and just being out in the sunshine and getting away from all thoughts of being overdue and looming inductions was probably what helped to get things going.

I woke up around 4am on Wednesday and noticed a slight dull ache around the bottom of my bump and upper thighs. I wasn't getting my hopes up that it would become anything more, but by the time we got up in the morning with the older girls it was still there and had got a bit stronger. With getting the girls up and dressed, pottering about the kitchen getting breakfast things out and so on, the aches had developed into regular waves which were coming and going, and I knew at this point we were heading in the right direction, but also had all the warnings in the back of my head that with third babies, early labour can stop and start and take a while to get going properly.

Chris took Hattie to school and I tidied up a bit in the kitchen while Martha played. When he got back the aching was becoming more regular, about every ten minutes but still very mild, so we agreed it would be worth ringing the homebirth team to let them know. Because the baby was measuring larger, Dani had said she would make sure they had two midwives for the birth (sometimes births are attended by a midwife and a maternity care assistant when things are likely to be straightforward), so they wanted to have plenty of notice to get the right people ready. As it turned out Dani was on leave that week, but had assured us that her colleagues were well briefed on my pregnancy so everything would be fine. We were told to call back when the contractions had got to one in ten minutes or were lasting more than 40 seconds. We rang my parents to ask them to come and collect Martha and the girls' overnight bags, and so by about 10.30 we were on our own in the house knowing that everyone *else was taken care of, so all we had to do was concentrate on having this baby!*

We had a cup of tea and watched some TV while I bounced on the ball, and Chris tidied up the playroom and moved toys out of the way to make the space a bit more relaxing! In a moment of excellent timing we took delivery of the girls' birthday present – a large outdoor trampoline – which could have arrived at any time that day – better than 4 hours later! I recall Chris making some comments about it helping to bring on labour but I wasn't convinced!

Sitting down didn't help with progress though (this is where we noticed the difference from the first two, that it could just slow down completely). The contractions got further apart and then more or less stopped. We had lunch and decided to go for a walk to get things moving, which definitely worked! We were out for about an hour and in that time the contractions ramped up a lot, coming much more frequently, and by the time we got back they were up to one minute long every few minutes. I called Beth who was the midwife on call that afternoon to let her know, and she said she'd pick up the birth kit and come over to check how things were progressing.

Again contractions slowed down even though I was bouncing on the ball still, so I started pacing the house, walking up and down the stairs and doing more squats (I'd been advised by midwives and other third time mums that squats were the best way to keep the head low and in contact with the cervix to encourage dilation – they certainly did the trick!).

Beth arrived at about 3pm and found I was between 3 and 4cm dilated and said she would call the other midwives to join her and start setting up the kit. Chris got the pool inflated and started filling it. By 4pm the pool was ready, and as well as Beth we had another community midwife and a care assistant who was really keen to see a homebirth but kept missing them so

173

had come along to observe. They set up all the homebirth kit, including resuscitation equipment for the baby, and the all-important gas and air!

In contrast to the first two labours, when I had found it really uncomfortable to stand and just wanted to be sitting bouncing on the birth ball, this time all I wanted to do was walk! When I mentioned I was getting tired walking all the time, someone suggested I tried the ball, but sitting on it this time was just like sitting on needles! So, I paced around the kitchen and up and down the room, stopping to lean on a wall or a chair for each contraction: I found it so helpful to lean on something and sway my hips or push back against the wall.

I tried each time to picture the golden thread as I was breathing through them. The back door was open into the garden cos it was so warm, and it was a gorgeous sunny day. I will always remember leaning on the back of a chair in the kitchen, imagining the golden thread stretching out down the garden outside. I came back to that image each time and it really helped me ride the contractions as they peaked and subsided. I almost felt like I was watching the contractions coming past like a line on a graph, I could see them coming, going up and then dropping away again. I don't remember feeling them in that way with either of the first two.

The other thing that was different was that I really didn't get on with the TENS machine this time round either. With the other two I'd found it helped a lot – it's so interesting how each labour is different, which shows that you really don't know what you will want or how you will react until you're in the middle of it. I suppose that also means that you can't guess how a subsequent birth will go, there's no reason it will follow the same pattern as the first, either for good or bad: you just have to take each one as a different experience.

When Beth said it was ok for me to get in the pool that was

a huge relief, the warmth of the water was incredible, and I was so ready for the gas and air by then too! But I think the relaxation of getting in the pool, plus from last time my body was clearly thinking, "When I get in the pool it's time to have a baby", meant the contractions stepped up a notch again! I kept remembering to try and keep my jaw loose as I was breathing on the Entonox, even if the breathing out wasn't quite so calm and quiet anymore! This time with the experience of two births behind me, I could even recognise myself going through the 'transition phase'. When I started telling Chris I couldn't do it, that I wanted to give up, I could almost sense the knowing looks around the room as they knew we were nearly there!

Then there was one contraction which was different, I felt the 'pop' of my waters breaking and the weight of the baby shifted. The Entonox had made me quite lightheaded by this point, and it sounded like Beth was far away when she was telling me to try and push slowly as the head came out. In the end I don't think I did any conscious pushing at all, I just let it happen, and while I was thinking 'It's never going to fit, I can't do it', I also knew from last time that it was so nearly there, which kept me going. Once the head was out, I had completely forgotten about all the worries about shoulder dystocia and large babies getting stuck, I just heard Beth behind me saying when the next one comes you just need one more push.

It felt like there was a pause as everything stopped, then I could feel it coming, and with one last push she was here. I caught her under the water and lifted her up, we rubbed her back to get her breathing, and Chris looked and said, 'I think we've got another girl!'. She was tangled in the cord round both arms, so needed a bit of unwrapping! We sat and looked at each other for a few minutes, completely amazed that I'd done it, again, before Chris cut the cord and I was helped out of the pool.

Chris did skin-to-skin with her while I was settled on the sofa to birth the placenta, which came away incredibly smoothly

175

compared to the first two, and then after that I needed a few stitches, although much less than with either of the other two despite her size! After that she came to me for a feed, having been rooting for milk on Chris the whole time, and once latched on, she kept going for over an hour! The midwives had another cup of tea and finished their notes, and then packed up their stuff while Chris emptied and deflated the pool. By 8.30 the midwives had all gone home, Chris put the pizza in the oven, and I went to have a shower.

It turned out the scans and measurements were right, she was 9lbs 4oz, and her head was over the 98th centile: pretty much what had been predicted, and not a small feat for a homebirth with minimal pain relief! Who says you can't have a big baby at home?!

Chris shares his perspective of the three births

Chris came to the birth preparation workshop with Sarah as a refresher before the birth of their third child. Often you get a glimpse of how a couple will work together during the birth journey and Chris seemed to me to be the solid rock that you would need; quietly watchful and ready to respond.

Hattie's birth:

I suppose I should feel like a bit of an expert as father/husband/ birth partner after the birth of three babies. But it's definitely true when people say that every birth is different.

The birth of our eldest, Hattie, was pretty much a textbook example of how a first birth should go. Sarah started to feel the beginnings of contractions mid-morning and gradually got stronger as the day went on. We went for a walk in the park and I started doing practical things like making sure the cat had food in case we were gone for a while. As Sarah's contractions ramped up over the afternoon, I double checked the hospital bag against our list and put on something lowbrow on TV to distract Sarah as she bounced away on her birth ball.

I also started religiously tracking how long and far apart her contractions were on an app, waiting until they hit the thresholds the hospital had set for coming in. In hindsight the day and early evening felt like it passed really quickly but I'm not sure it felt like that at the time. Eventually Sarah's contractions were sufficiently far apart and we put bags into the car and headed to the hospital. My only memory of the drive is Sarah being really unimpressed at going round roundabouts mid-contraction but there wasn't really much choice!

After one false start where we were sent home again, we were put in a room in the delivery suite with an inflatable birth pool because the midwife-led unit was full. This was the first of many times during all three labours where I thought I might need to advocate for the birth experience that I knew Sarah wanted but, as with all the other times, the midwives were one step ahead of me – when they said Sarah had to go to the delivery suite, they'd already arranged the birth pool and reassured Sarah that it would be a midwife-led delivery.

The next three hours or so are a bit of a blur – my only real memory was sore knees from kneeling next to the birth pool for hours on end (which Sarah has pointed out was considerably less discomfort than she was experiencing!). When it came to pushing, Sarah experienced the classic 'transition' where she felt like she couldn't go on. This was the first time (again something which happened at all three births) where I got a reassur-

ing knowing look from the midwife that said everything was ok and my job was to reassure Sarah and keep going.

After what felt like a very long hour, and eventually with some encouragement and directing from the midwife, Sarah pushed out our daughter. Every time I look back at photos of those first five minutes, I remember the mix of dazed amazement both at what Sarah had done and the tiny little life that we had.

After some stiches, weighing and Sarah getting multiple coverings with baby poo, we went up to the post-natal ward. By now it was early morning and once Sarah was settled, I had to go home until visiting hours. While the uninterrupted sleep that day and the following night was appreciated, the 48 hours that followed where Sarah was kept in and I had to go home out of visiting hours made me feel totally helpless because Sarah was left in without me to help overnight because Hattie struggled to breastfeed. This formed a large part of our decision about how and where to have our next baby.

Martha's birth:

We'd had a discussion before Hattie was born about having a homebirth with future babies but Sarah's experience of feeling alone and isolated on the postnatal ward made us even more sure we wanted to do it. So, two years later, when baby number two was on the way, we started conversations with our midwives about having the baby at home. This felt like a bit of a battle at times: Sarah's notes from the first birth mentioned having a certain level of blood loss (which no-one mentioned to us at the time), which meant our community midwife wouldn't commit to a homebirth without talking to the consultant midwife. Which took weeks. But, eventually, we started making plans to have a baby at home. We borrowed a pool from the local homebirth group, borrowed towels from lots of people and lots of other things that people recommended that we did. The *birth started much like the others – Sarah had some back ache which gave me a hint that I should work from home rather than have to rush back. And after a morning trip to the park with Hattie, backache turned into contractions. So, Hattie went to Sarah's parents, I inflated the pool and Sarah sat bouncing on a birth ball in front of the TV for distraction.*

When I rang the hospital after lunch, we were told that they could only support a homebirth until 7pm because they didn't have experienced staff on overnight. We tried to put that to the back of our minds and just see how labour progressed and, sure enough, in an hour or so Sarah's contractions had reached the level where we would have gone into hospital. The hospital arranged for a midwife to come and see us (we later learnt she came midway through her community clinic at our local children's centre).

I filled the pool (including a hilarious moment where I was boiling multiple pans and kettles because the water tank emptied) while Sarah bounced on her ball. When the midwife arrived, after a quick examination which showed Sarah was just about in active labour, Sarah hopped into the pool. The midwife said that a colleague would be along soon and would bring some gas and air for when things ramped up.

No sooner had the midwife sat down at our kitchen table to start writing some notes, Sarah suddenly started to feel the urge to push. The midwife only had to look at Sarah to tell that she was fully dilated and ready to push: a massive shock to both of us. The midwife went to her car and came back with a bin bag full of equipment that she carried in her boot. Sarah got worried that it was all happening before she was expecting it to but, as before, the midwife reassured us that sometimes this happens.

As the baby's head started to come out, the midwife's mood shifted: she went from being friendly and chatty to very fo-

cused. Luckily Sarah didn't spot it but I realised that she wasn't expecting to be delivering a baby on her own. After not very long, Sarah pushed out another baby girl. Less than an hour after the midwife arrived and three hours before the shift change that had worried us earlier! And I had exactly the same amazed feeling that I had the first time. Ten minutes or so later, I opened to door to a care assistant with gas and air and then a second midwife. Both were pretty shocked when I came to the door with a newborn baby!

But then the amazing bit of having a homebirth happened. After Sarah and the baby had been examined, midwives had written their notes and I'd cleared up the pool, everyone went home. And we were left in our house with just us and our new daughter. We put a pizza in the oven and enjoyed getting to know Martha.

Isabel's birth:

After that brilliant experience, we had no hesitation in arranging a homebirth three years later when Sarah was pregnant again. Since our last baby, a dedicated homebirth team had been established so there was no worry about whether there'd be anyone on shift. And it meant Sarah had all her antenatal appointments at home. Like the first time, we had a slight battle to have Sarah cleared for homebirth: the baby measured big and scans showed that Sarah had more fluid than normal.

But by the time the baby came to full term, the fluid levels had gone down and we'd decided (admittedly against an obstetrician's advice) to stick to a homebirth. The homebirth midwife team couldn't have been more supportive and I joined a conversation about exactly how they'd deal with the complications that can come with delivering a large baby and how little that differed to what they'd do in hospital.

Sarah's third labour began much like the first two: backache *that gradually ramped up over the course of a morning. Our eldest was at school and we sent three-year-old Martha to Sarah's parents. Unfortunately, Sarah's midwife was on holiday, but she'd told us who to expect in her absence. The contractions took a little longer to build up than with Martha so after lunch, we decided to go for a walk in the woods near our house. Over the course of 30 minutes or so, Sarah got to the point where contractions were coming thick and fast (we had to try and avoid people on the way home so we didn't scare them with a very large pregnant woman having quite substantial contractions on the street!).*

We called the midwife and she came around with an incredible amount of equipment. In contrast to Martha's birth when we only had a bin bag of essential kit; this time we saw what we should have had! There were boxes and bags full of stuff. Gas and air, oxygen, a fully set-up resus station for the baby, and much, much more. And before too long, a second midwife and a care assistant. It felt like our house was a mini-hospital!

As is apparently normal with third babies, labour progressed a bit more slowly and stop-start than with the other two. I felt like a bit of a spare part for the next couple of hours. Sarah was most comfortable when pacing about and was very focused, so I stuck to making tea for midwives, topping up the pool with warm water and being a leaning post for Sarah from time to time. The midwives sat discreetly timing contractions on their watches and reassuring Sarah that everything was progressing as it should.

Eventually, Sarah wanted to get into the pool and I assumed the familiar position kneeling by the edge of the pool. This time I could at least offer her gas and air. As with the first two, Sarah had a very obvious transition point where she started saying that she couldn't do it – but this time I think even she could tell that was actually a positive sign that things were progressing. The most amazing thing for me this time was that, thanks to a

*specially purchased large mirror, I watched our baby's head be-
ing slowly pushed out. And then suddenly, with one more push,
Sarah had a baby in her arms – yet another girl!*

*This time I had some skin-to-skin with the baby while Sarah de-
livered the placenta and was stitched up. And then, after all the
notes were written, the baby had been weighed and I'd cleared
up the pool, we were again left alone in our own home to get to
know our newest baby.*

*I know that in lots of ways we were fortunate – neither Sarah
nor the baby had any health issues in any of the pregnancies
or labours. But I am left with such a positive memory of the
births of our daughters. We had three amazing midwives who
combined clinical skill, a real respect for the birth experience
that we wanted and an amazing calm reassurance that gave us
confidence that everything would be ok. But most of all, Sarah
did what came naturally to her and each time (mostly) calmly
focused on birthing our baby. I don't have words to express my
admiration for how she did that.*

It is so wonderful to hear the father's voice and see some differences in detail about the births. What I always appreciated about
Sarah when she was in my classes is that she does her research,
makes her decision and then is at peace. It takes confidence to go
against the advice of a consultant, but it's worth thinking about
what the norm is for each health professional that you encounter.
If you are surrounded daily by challenging births because of existing medical conditions on the delivery suite, you are more likely to
recommend a hospital birth. If you attend homebirths daily, supporting physiological birth, you will be confident in recommending those for normal, healthy pregnancies (even of big babies).

Ultimately, the parents of the baby need to decide what is right for them after understanding the issues, weighing up the statistics and following their intuition about what will support the mother to feel safe. Once safety has been established comes the opportunity to enter into a quiet confidence and inner stillness as you approach the birth (with, on the surface, the quite normal roller-coaster of emotions that happen as hormones increase as you get closer to your birth journey).

BOX 14: Three-minute mindfulness practice: the body scan

Take a deep breath and prepare to scan through your body. Start at the head and pay attention to anything you feel. If there is a sensation, it might trigger a thought or emotion, but try to return to the scan of sensations, moving onto the neck and shoulders. Keep taking your awareness down through the body, observing any sensations (they might include an itch, warmth, coldness, hunger, aching, heaviness, giddiness). Take your attention down one arm at a time, to the hands and fingers. Give particular presence of mind to the chest and belly: often our emotions show up here as sensations (for example, tightness, warmth, expansion, butterflies, clenching). Continue down one leg at a time, to the feet and toes. Remember the back of the body, including the buttocks.

Often the sensations will pass by themselves as you take a few more breaths, but if needed you can respond. For example, going to the toilet to relieve that urge to wee that you've had for an hour. Or stretching when you realise there is tension from sitting still for too long.

Some of you may have found this book with a subsequent pregnancy, having had a first birth that did not go how you had hoped. This may have been because you did not realise the preparation required or perhaps you prepared as fully as you could have, but some unexpected situation derailed your birth journey. With the benefit of hindsight, you may realise that some aspect of how to create this cocoon of safety was missing. Perhaps a birth doula will give you the reassurance that someone experienced in birth can advocate for your needs or an appointment with a consultant midwife can lead to a document to outline your specific wishes or situation. Reflecting on how your body responded in the first birth can give you clues as to what to change in the lead up to this next birth. Spending time reflecting on how to make this pregnancy and birth different can transform the journey and heal previous experiences.

Affirmations (Box 15) can be a positive way to create an empowering feedback loop in relation to the birth and a quietness of mind. I have a wonderful memory of a friend, Carine, who gave birth to her second child at home. I went around to their house 11 hours after her son was born to congratulate them as no family were nearby. In every room, there was the same birth affirmation written on card and stuck to different things: the cupboard in the kitchen, the mantel piece in the lounge, the mirror in the bathroom: "I trust my body to birth my baby". The dad joked that even he trusted his body to birth the baby after so many months of looking at these affirmations. She also had the flower wreath from her mother blessing hanging in the lounge where the baby was born.

BOX 15: Birth Affirmations

You can find a list of affirmations based on this book at www.pearlsofbirthwisdom.com. However, it can be powerful to create your own based on what you most need to hear. When creating your own, the sentence should be in the present tense and positively phrased, such as "Every breath gets me closer to meeting my baby". Avoid negatives as your brain will latch on to the verb and ignore the qualifier. For example, "I will not be afraid of the contractions" will focus the brain on the fear.

You may decide to have a range of affirmations that you put around your home or on your screensaver at work, or you may have a particular affirmation that sums up how you want to feel through the birth journey that you put everywhere. One of my favourites to use in class is the simple "All is well". Particularly if you struggle with anxious thoughts or catastrophising, work to use the affirmation like a mantra that you repeat to focus the mind on the possibility of things going well (and seek external support if needed).

It may seem paradoxical, but all of the preparation and reflection encouraged by this book to create a cocoon of safety is to facilitate an allowing and a letting go of control. To be comfortable to do this, we control as much as we can beforehand: for example, staying active during pregnancy, preparing our birth plan so we know the birth partner is primed for advocacy, practicing relaxation techniques so we can calm our nervous systems, choosing the location for the birth carefully. Then the greatest task during birth is to physically and emotionally let go of this baby that has grown inside and been protected for nine months or more. We also have to let go of our ideas of how our birth should be and let our bodies and our unique situations guide us.

A good analogy for this is pottery! When I was doing my PhD, I went to pottery class to spend time doing something tactile and creative. I could only control the creative process so far though: I created the shape of the pot as I wanted it, chose the glazes and trusted the technician to set the right temperature of the kiln for firing. Once you put your pot in the kiln and walked away, you never knew exactly what the piece would look like when it was done firing, as the glaze could turn out in unexpected ways. This is also good preparation for parenting, because although you may imagine your child to be a particular way (perhaps a mini version of you), they grow up in their own unique way and you can only support them in that! Parenting is a constant process of letting go of your expectations and attachments.

📖 REFLECTIONS ⟩ on Stillness

If I asked you to be still for 15 minutes, I wonder what your reaction be: a gladness to stop and simply be or alarm that you were wasting time perhaps? The questions below are guiding you towards finding a quality of stillness as you approach the birth of your baby.

When you think about the upcoming birth, is there anything remaining that worries you or feels unfinished? What steps can you take to feel more positive?

What messages do you override from your body? (E.g. the urge to go to the toilet, an aching pelvis when walking a lot later in pregnancy, the need for a nap when the nursery needs painting) What commitment will you make to your body today to respect the signals she's giving you?

What helps you personally to be mindful and present? (E.g. Golden Thread Breath (Box 1), Resting Breath (Box 4), Listening to the Body (Box 6), Body Scan (Box 14) or paying attention to your body as you do yoga, swimming or other movement)

What message do you most need to hear now? How can you turn it into an affirmation to repeat inside your head in times of doubt, or to put around your home where you can see it repeatedly?

SUGGESTIONS

Make an intention to do five minutes of mindfulness meditation a day.

Choose an activity to do with awareness and presence of mind. It may be eating the first five mouthfuls of your lunch or paying attention to your surroundings as you take a walk rather than being distracted by thoughts.

Put your affirmations onto cards and put them around your home where you'll see them often.

RESOURCES

The Mindfulness App – for finding an inner quiet

www.mbct.co.uk or *www.bemindfulonline.com* (Take a Mindfulness course based on Cognitive Behavioural Therapy to have a way of managing anxieties if they keep surfacing.)

Jane Hardwicke Collings (2007) *Ten Moons: The Inner Journey of Pregnancy, Preparation for Natural Birth*. Lulu.com

Pearl 9
Vulnerability

*When it is safe to be vulnerable,
it is powerful beyond measure.
Vulnerability allows us to move
into a new level of trusting and
connecting deeply with others.*

Imagine how the birthing journey has been unfolding. The midwife says that she can see the baby's head and you are soon to meet your child. Your birth partner was reluctant to see the baby actually emerging from your vulva or to cut the cord, but in the process of the journey, has witnessed your strength and the female body's incredible capacity, and cannot take their eyes away from witnessing this miracle of life. Your vulnerability during this rite of passage has humbled them and they want to be part of this journey by cutting the umbilical cord so that one day they can say that the incredible moment when mother and child became two separate entities, they were right there.

Vulnerability in our culture is often seen as a weakness and we often make decisions to ensure that we are not vulnerable. However, being vulnerable in a safe situation allows us to deepen our connection with others. During the birthing journey we become physically vulnerable because the surges take all of our focus and, if in fact we do not feel safe, the body shuts down the contractions so that we can respond accordingly. However, there is a deeper physical vulnerability at work because that intimate part of ourselves is opening incredibly. It is possible for the cervix to close up and to become less dilated than before, when something or someone intrudes on the journey.

Emotionally, birth requires courage to be vulnerable, particularly the first time when we do not know what our reaction to birthing will be physically or emotionally. The transition between the first stage of labour (the thinning and opening of the cervix) and the second stage (the baby moving down and out) is a classic time when vulnerability may show up. Commonly the mother will say things like, "I've had enough of this, let's go home" or, "I didn't sign up for this, I'm not doing it anymore" or, "Do we really want a baby anyway?". Out of context, these statements seem silly, even illogical, but it is a call to witness her at the edge of her known experience in this liminal space. Transition is often more emotionally intense for first births, which some say is because the woman's identity is about to shift. Seeing transition from this lens, a woman who says "I can't do it" is right. She (the woman who has never had a child) cannot do it, but the mother she is becoming *can*. Once the fears of leaving behind her old identity fade, she can move into the last phase of pregnancy, give birth, and become the mother her baby needs.

From a physiological perspective, transition is when the uterus is changing what she is doing: from using the long muscles to open the cervix to using the round muscles to squeeze the baby down like toothpaste out of a tube!* Women can feel this change in their bodies and can panic if they don't know what is happening. However, when the pushing starts it can feel wonderful and renew the focus. For some mothers, transition does not manifest like this at all, but appears as a time to "rest and be thankful". Contractions may fade as the uterus reorganises herself and the intelligent body has a chance to rest before the final push (forgive the pun!). This mother may find her vulnerable point comes at a different time and the safety created by the birth partner or the midwife allows her to grow into a new level of emotional maturity and trust. It's quite normal to have a wobble and this may be a sign that labour has entered a new phase.

(*There are three sets of muscles in the uterus: the long, round and spiral muscles. The latter are what turn the baby to bring the head and shoulders through the pelvis. The uterus isn't symmetrical as shown in most of the images I've ever seen, but straighter on the right-hand side. This asymmetry can help the baby nestle their back in the mum's left-hand side, which is curved.)

Read Rebecca's story of vulnerability next.

REBECCA'S BIRTHING STORY

(homebirth, hospital transfer)

Rebecca is a young woman in her twenties and an engineer. She made me laugh a lot during the pregnancy yoga classes, and later the mother and baby ones, with her deadpan manner when recounting funny events.

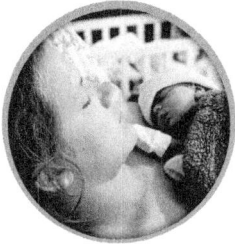

Matilda's Birth:

My contractions started at four in the morning on Friday 23rd of August. I remember the first one being like the Braxton Hicks I had been experiencing for the previous week, but this one was accompanied with a period pain like sensation. I remember it was over quite quickly and almost immediately I was convincing myself that it couldn't possibly be a contraction. About 20 minutes later I started to get the same feeling, and again once it was over, I convinced myself again that it couldn't possibly be a contraction. The third time that this happened, I accepted that I was in labour.

Sam started to stir, so I asked him if he was ok. He said he was fine and asked me how I was, and I replied, "Think I'm in labour." He spun over instantly to make sure that I was ok and asked how I was feeling. I felt fine, the contractions didn't hurt at all, they were just like normal period pain sensations that I experienced all the time.

By this time, it was about five in the morning, and so we decided that as we weren't going to be going back to sleep anytime soon, we may as well get up and have some breakfast. I had a homebirth planned and so the lounge downstairs had been set up for the last three weeks with towels, sheets, the hired birth pool, a hot stone to diffuse essential oils, a homemade washing line across the middle of the lounge with baby clothes hanging off of it for inspiration to get through the labour, and of course my birth plan.

We had breakfast and then went into the lounge where we decided that the television would stay off, a Spotify playlist of Hypnobirthing music would play, and I would move around the lounge assuming various positions learnt from pregnancy yoga. For most of the morning these positions included lying on my side with my pregnancy pillow, being on all fours and swirling my hips around, and bouncing on my ball.

We got to about 1pm and the intensity of the contractions had increased only slightly. From breakfast onwards the contractions had been every 10 to 15 minutes and weren't even painful enough to have to breathe through. At about this time Sam decided to head out to the shop to get some food for dinner. He left and I didn't have a contraction for the entire 35 minutes that he was away for. As soon as the car rolled onto the drive, I started having another contraction. This absolutely fascinated both of us, as we had done the birth preparation workshop and were very attuned to the importance of oxytocin during labour.

At about 4pm I was [sitting] on the ball and I said to Sam that we should probably let the homebirth team midwives know that I was in labour. I phoned Gemma and told her that my contractions were every ten minutes or so and that the pain was manageable but that I wanted to let her know so that I was on her radar. She told me to carry on as I was as I seem to be cop-ing well, and to let her know when I was three to five minutes apart or if my waters broke.

As the evening wore on the contractions started to get a bit more intense. By about 8pm, the position that was working for [me] the most was the knotted scarf over the door trick that Tessa had told me. As the contraction got more intense I would sit more deeply into a squat, while hanging off the door as Sam pushed on my sacrum. By 10pm Sam was basically asleep, and I was very tired but unable to sleep as the contractions were still every ten minutes. I suggested that we go upstairs and try and get some sleep as we had been up for 16 hours and the worst was still to come.

Sam was asleep before his head hit the pillow. Unfortunately, my contractions were now painful enough and still every ten minutes so I was unable to get any sleep. I tried stacking my pillows up in a tall tower and leaning on them on the bed. I tried sleeping on my side, but this was very painful when I had a contraction. I tried kneeling on the floor and leaning my head on the bed, but nothing worked. I decided to have a bath to see if that would slow it down or speed it up. I didn't want to fill up the birth pool until I was in established labour. The bath was the worst decision I made all night. During the labour so far, I had had the freedom to move about and assume any position that felt comfortable during the contraction. In the bath I was stuck on my back and felt trapped. I abandoned this idea after about half an hour and went downstairs again, leaving Sam in bed.

By this point it was after midnight and the contractions were very strong. For about an hour I was kneeling on two cushions on the floor, and had my head and arms leaning on the sofa. The contractions were still every ten minutes apart and I was starting to reach the upper boundary of my pain threshold. At 1am on Saturday morning, I went back upstairs and woke Sam up. I told him that I couldn't do it without him anymore and

193

I really needed him to coach my breathing and help massage my back. We went back downstairs and almost immediately, my contractions sped up to every three to five minutes. I called Gemma the midwife, and after having several contractions on the phone to her, she decided to come and see me.

Gemma arrived at the house around 2am and monitored me as I had contractions. They were still every three to five minutes and were very strong. I was now leaning over the arm of the sofa [with] Sam pushing strongly on my sacrum as I had a contraction. Despite the pain being very intense now, I was still very calm and happy between them. I was laughing and joking and as soon as the contraction is over was in the mindset that I could conquer the next one. In the gaps between them, Sam would run between the kitchen and the lounge, checking on the hose and water temperature to fill up the birth pool. At one point I told everyone that I felt sick, and as soon as Sam put a bucket in front of me, I was sick.

After this my enthusiasm and determination started to wane. I was absolutely shattered and now didn't have any energy. This was at about 3am and the birth pool was full and ready. Gemma did a vaginal examination and told me that I was only 3 to 4cm. I was very wary about getting into the birth pool because I didn't want my contractions to get further apart, as to me this meant that my labour would be going backwards. Gemma told me that I clearly needed rest and that the birth pool would either speed the labour up to the point where I was giving birth [or] slow labour down and allow me to get some much-needed rest. I knew she was right and I knew that I had to listen to my body.

I got into the birth pool and was immediately relieved. The warm water felt good and my contractions went back up to eight to ten minutes apart, which allowed me to relax a little. Around 4am Gemma decided to leave and go home, as I was managing the contractions well and they hadn't shown any sign of speeding up. Between contractions I would rest my head in Sam's hands and try and get some sleep. Gemma left and the contractions increased in intensity. I remember my breathing getting less controlled and started to make moaning sounds instead. Sam managed to guide me back to breathing and we continued like this until 5.30am.

At this time, I suddenly felt like I needed to go for a poo. The contractions were still every ten minutes or so, and despite being given a sieve to use in the event of pooing in the pool, I knew I was capable of getting to the toilet and preferred to do so. Sam helps me out of the pool and upstairs to the loo. Whilst on the toilet I had a contraction, vomited, and had a poo. I was completely done at this point. This wasn't fair. I knew that I was going to have to push a baby out of me, but I didn't sign up for vomiting and pooing at the same time. Having a contraction while being sick and having a poo is honestly one of the most painful things I have ever experienced. I told Sam that I was giving up and wasn't going to do this anymore.

Thankfully Sam had been paying a lot of attention in the NCT classes and birth preparation workshop, as he turned round to me and said, "Rebecca this sounds like transition and I think we're getting closer." I realised he was right, but I was in so much pain. This is where I said to him that I wanted gas and air. He fully informed me that the midwives weren't with us and neither was the gas and air and that I would have to carry on doing what I was doing. We got back downstairs and got back into the birth pool and about 20 minutes later I realised I wanted another poo.

I was so tired and so frustrated but still was not keen to poo in the pool. We went back upstairs and much to my joy, had another contraction while vomiting again. I sat there waiting for the poo to finish this joyous occasion. However, the poo did not come. I remember my tiredness subsiding immediately and looking at Sam with full awareness that I needed to push.

195

This could not be happening.
I was every ten minutes still.
The midwives were not with us.
I was on the toilet for goodness sake.
In that moment my birth plan disintegrated.

I got off the loo and used a sink to push against. Sam was on the phone to Gemma and my breathing had gone out the window. I didn't feel like I was having normal contractions anymore – it was just constant pain. Gemma said that she thought I was probably about to have the baby and was on her way. I remember shouting at the top of my lungs, "Make her bring the gas and air!".

Gemma said she would have to stop by the hospital to get this but would be there as soon as possible (we live five minutes from the hospital). Meanwhile the urge to push had intensified and I was terrified that I was going to poo myself and so returned to the toilet. I sat on the loo and knew that I had to push. I was scared because midwives weren't with us.

I remember distinctly saying to Sam, "No one is here".
Sam very calmly looked at me and said, "I'm here."
And this was all I needed.

I knew that midwives or no midwives, Sam was going to be here for me.

I wanted to fight the urge to push though and so I put my hand between my legs as if to stop myself from weeing. I was immediately terrified when I did this. I could feel what I thought was my baby's head. I remember holding myself and the sensation of trying to not poo.

At about 6.30am Gemma arrived at the house. I was still on the toilet holding my baby in, and she very calmly appeared at the top of the stairs on my landing and asked me if I was ok. She saw that I was holding myself and asked was I holding myself because it felt comfortable or because I was holding something back. I told her both.

She told me that she thought I was probably quite close to having my baby and could she convince me to get off the toilet? I managed to get onto all fours just in front of the toilet and Gemma snuck between the toilet and me and had a look.

She said very simply, yep they are the membranes. You're about to have a baby.

My waters hadn't broken and she explained that initially I would be pushing to pop them. She told me that I was safe, that she was there, and that I could now trust my body and push. So I did.

The sensation of pushing was unlike anything I have ever experienced in my life. It started off feeling a bit like having a poo, but then just kept growing and growing in intensity. After about two sets of pushes I begged Gemma to let me have the gas and air. She told me that it wasn't going to do anything for the pain as I was too far along, but that it might be a nice distraction. I took the mouthpiece between my teeth and despite desperately trying not to bite down on it, but did anyway.

After a couple more pushes my waters popped. Gemma told me that the baby was going to be here soon and did I want to move as this would be my last chance. I said yes, and I knew that we wouldn't be able to get downstairs to the birth pool, so Sam quickly went and got the waterproof tarp from downstairs and laid it over the bed.

In the next gap between pushes, Sam helped me onto a bed where I assumed an all-fours position and buried my head in my pillows. I listened to Gemma and pushed when she told me to. I remember the feeling of the pushing urge fading and being upset that the baby still hasn't been born, and knowing that that meant I was going to have to push again. But I knew that my body was doing what it needed to and that if I had to push again, I had to push again.

Gemma asked if [Sam] wanted to come and have a look at our baby being born, and much to Sam's horror, he informed Gemma that he didn't need to move as our full-length mirrors on our wardrobes were giving him the full show. (Sam told me after this that he wouldn't have had it any other way and that watching our baby come into this world was the best thing that he had ever seen.)

At 7.01am on Saturday the 24th of August, Matilda was born into this world. I would have gotten away with everything scot free if she hadn't have come out with her little hand on her cheek. Thankfully she left my perineum intact but unfortunately this little hand took a notch out of the side as she came out.

I was absolutely shattered. I remember leaning onto my heels, looking up at the ceiling as if to finally breathe now that I had given birth. Then Gemma said, "Rebecca look down and pick up your baby". I looked down and there was this tiny 6lb 8oz little thing staring up at me. I picked her up and gave her a cuddle and remember just being completely amazed and utterly flabbergasted at the whole thing.

After about five minutes of being in this position, Sam cutting the cord and both of us having a little cry, I was told, could I have a cough? A little confused, I obliged. Apparently, my placenta was right there ready to come out. I had opted for a physiological third stage and had been prepared for it to last up to an hour. After a couple more coughs and then lying on my back, I deliver the placenta nine minutes after birth.

Unfortunately, I started losing a bit too much blood and they asked if they could give me the injection. I have a phobia of needles and despite just having a baby was absolutely terrified to accept. I started to panic, and they said ok we'll give you a little longer and see if you stop bleeding. A couple of minutes later, I hadn't, and they said they really wanted to give me the injection. I accepted. And cried.

They made sure that all of the placenta was there and I thought that I was done. Unfortunately, where her hand had been on her face, and where she torn the side of my vagina, I need to have stitches. I remember taking advantage of the gas and air, and after half an hour was stitched up.

They took me to the loo for a wee and cleaned me up a bit before letting me return to bed to finally relax.

Every time I've read this story, I cry at the point where Sam says, "I'm here." That is the cocoon of safety I've been writing about in this book encapsulated into one moment. To choose to be vulnerable with someone requires courage and daring. During birth we are not always able to choose whether to be vulnerable or not, it happens anyway because of the nature of this intense physical and emotional rite of passage. Where a woman is not prepared for this, it can feel shocking or traumatic. Or it may push her into a new and positive experience of vulnerability depending on how the birth journey plays out. Preferably everyone in the room is prepared to some degree for supporting the labouring woman and can rise to the occasion.

KATE'S BIRTHING STORY

(hospital birth during COVID-19 crisis)

As I was finishing writing the book, the pandemic occurred and anxiety levels were high because maternity policies changed significantly. One of the most worrying issues for expectant mums was the fact that not all hospitals were allowing birth partners to come into hospital at all, while others limited attendance to one birth partner during active labour and only as long as they had no symptoms of the virus. Kate was putting a brave face on the situation, but I knew she was worried about the practicalities of care for her first child during labour and her parents not be able to help postnatally.

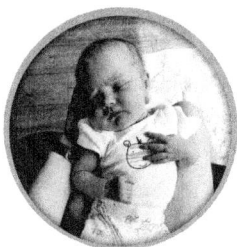

Percy's Birth:

Our due date was Sunday 26th April...a date that came and went with little event. By the evening of Tuesday 28th, I had begun to have the odd twinge, but went to bed as usual. By the morning, I woke having contractions regularly but only about ten minutes apart.

My parents and my family of three had all been self-isolating in the lead up to the birth. We decided that we had to technically 'break the rules,' sending my daughter, Martha, into the care of grandparents, but we viewed it as an 'essential' trip as she had to go somewhere!

We decided to get our daughter to her grandparents in case we needed to get to hospital. Martha went to Granny and Grandad's and I decided to try to sleep. I woke after a couple of hours and the contractions had pretty much completely stopped. We spent the afternoon watching box sets and wondering when our baby might arrive!

By about 6pm that evening, Martha came home and we got her to bed after tea. By 9pm, it all kicked off again, but again fairly slowly (contractions approximately eight to nine minutes apart).

We decided to go to bed to try to get some rest in the comfort of our own home. It wasn't the most peaceful lie down in the world (!), but we had music on and I was able to breathe through the contractions using the Golden Thread Breath we had practised.

At home, I spent quite a bit of time leaning over the ball and lying on my side in bed with cushions whilst resting.

By midnight, the contractions were more frequent, now about every six minutes, so Jack rang triage. It sounded like they were having a quiet night on the delivery suite and so would be happy to see us.

We called Jack's mum and she came to our house to stay over with Martha. We got to hospital about 1.30am to find I was about 6cm dilated. Jack had to wait outside the room while I was assessed, due to the COVID-19 risk (he should have actually stayed outside the hospital in the car but there was a mix up!) Once it was clear we were going to go home with a baby, Jack was allowed back into the room and we made our way to the delivery suite.

201

Whilst in an ideal world we would have preferred to have been on the midwife-led Rushey ward (which was closed due to COVID-19), the delivery room was private, with its own bathroom, and we were able to adjust the lighting and furniture for a comfortable environment. The midwives read our birth plan in detail and also helped foster a calm atmosphere whilst I laboured.

In Rushey, where I had my first baby, the beds change into all sorts of positions, so I think I spent most of my [first] labour kneeling and on the birth pool with Martha. That wasn't really possible this time, as it was just a fairly standard bed, but I think if you go in prewarned, you can still adapt the space as best you can [and] make a comfortable birthing environment.

At 4.26am, Percy was born with just deep breathing and gas and air to assist. I delivered on my back, which was what the midwife advised – not what I imagined, but all was well. By that point, I just needed the baby out! I ended up having an episiotomy like last time, I think more for precaution so that I didn't tear, and once stitched back up again, we remained in the delivery suite and awaited discharge from the midwives.

We were told we could go more or less straight home or I could stay in for the day with Percy while Jack went home (also due to the COVID risk). We opted for the former. The midwives obviously checked [that] both baby and I were fit and well before we were discharged, but it is a positive of the current situation that all parties want you home as soon as possible.

Before heading home, I was also offered a non-obligatory COVID-19 nasal and throat test. This fortunately came back negative!

It is a really difficult time for everyone at the moment, whether you're pregnant or not. Whilst it may not be what you were hoping for, my advice would be only focus on the things you can control. Positive energy is what gets you through the labour.

Yes, the midwives wore face masks and looked different, but they still took great care of me.

Percy was 7lb 14oz.

I have been relieved to hear many positive experiences from women who have given birth during the COVID-19 crisis. The midwives and all the other health professionals that I have heard about have been outstanding in their commitment to caring and have shown great empathy. Despite juggling a newborn and a toddler without her parents help, Kate was keen to share her experience to put others' minds at rest. Pregnancy and birth can feel like a vulnerable time anyway, but the global crisis has amplified this feeling of vulnerability many times over. It has been wonderful to see how much women want their birth partners at their side and that this has become the expected norm.

That said, it's relatively recent that men have been invited into the birth room. Not so long ago they would pace the corridor until news came. This means that many male partners very much want to have a hands-on role, but do not know explicitly what their role is or how they can be most helpfully supportive. When it becomes apparent that birth partners are not a spectator of the process but an active participant in the journey, they react in all sorts of ways. Sometimes there is anxiety that they will not have the confidence to be an advocate. Often, they become committed to practising techniques that they have been half-hearted about before. Occasionally, they realise that they themselves need support. Many of the techniques in the books are as much for the partner to stay calm, as they are for the birthing woman. Most times the birth partner is the most incredible source of support for the labouring woman. As such, birth partners frequently undertake their own internal journey into deeper maturity.

In the Red Tent women's circle that I facilitate, creating a safe space to be vulnerable and authentic is at the heart of what I do. I ask that the women are non-judgemental, maintain confidentiality and take responsibility for their feelings, asking for support when needed. When an opportunity for honest talk is created, women feel validated in all that they have experienced, and compassion and empathy flood the gathering.

What I have learnt over the five years of running the Red Tent so far, is that the more you allow yourself to be vulnerable, the greater connection you achieve with others. The barrier to vulnerability is shame. When we are afraid that others will judge us for how we behave, we shut down. Or when 'negative' emotions arise we may try to push them away. It is useful to prepare birth partners for the big emotions that often arise for the labouring woman during the birthing journey (Box 16). They often come at times when there is a shift in the labour and can be seen as a sign of things progressing well rather than something to be nervous of.

BOX 16: Feeling the feels

When reflecting on the questions below, or when you feel emotions arising over the next few weeks, see whether you can stay with the emotion until it changes. This is easy enough with the emotions we call positive like joy, love, excitement, but is harder with so-called negative emotions like sadness, irritation, anger or shame. When you notice the emotion, see if your tendency is to push it down, distract yourself or move into numbness. Sometimes secondary emotions like anger are masking other ones such as embarrassment or fear, so as you sit with one feeling, others may arise.

At a time when you are both relaxed and have time, ask your birth partner if they would agree to share how they honestly feel about the upcoming birth. Sometimes they want to protect you from their anxiety, but if you reassure them that you want to be as prepared as possible and want to listen, you may deepen your connection around the pregnancy and birth. You may need to share how you feel first to give them the confidence to reciprocate.

A couple of ground rules: 1) Listen without interruption – you'll have your turn. 2) Respect their feelings even if they do not accord with yours. 3) Leave solutions until later. Sometimes being listened to is enough to transform a feeling.

Being honest with yourself and your birth partner about what you're feeling and how you envision your birth can create a beautiful opportunity for connection. Spend time practising talking about your emotions and listening to your birth partner's unique journey. Also talk with your partner about the sounds you are likely to make in labour (Box 17). Vocalising can help us relax and let the sensations move through our bodies, but loud noises can be startling and scary for our partners if they are unprepared. As women, many of us have been taught to stay silent. Labour can be a beautiful part of the healing journey to reclaim your voice.

BOX 17: Using sound

The sounds that you make will change over the course of the birthing journey. Perhaps from a sigh as you focus on deeper breathing initially to a roar as the baby crowns. It is different for everyone but making sound can give you a focus through contractions and help you lean into the sensations.

Any sound that relaxes the throat area will have a knock-on positive effect to the pelvic floor to soften and open. Sounds like "Beuuuuuu", "Ahhhhh" or "Mmmmmm". As the baby moves down, the sound is likely to be stronger, like "GAAAAAA". Again, birth partners should see this as a welcome sign that things are progressing nicely rather than be alarmed! If they know this in advance, they can encourage you to get louder and louder if that helps you.

With preparation for this rite of passage, and positive external support, it can be a deepening into maturity. This can be gained in other ways for those that do not birth children, but I am particularly fascinated by the rites of passage that are in-built within our female bodies like menarche (first period), birth and menopause. After my births, I had a new respect for my body, my partner had frank admiration for what I had done, and I felt empowered. This is my hope for every woman.

📖 REFLECTIONS 〉 on Vulnerability

I would love you to revisit this section after the birth of your baby. Did your journey create a crucible for vulnerability to transform into empowerment? These reflections provide a space to trust in the process.

Write down what your most vulnerable moments have been. Can you describe vulnerable experiences that had positive outcomes too? What was the difference between the situations where vulnerability felt like a weakness and where it felt like a strength and created greater connection?

How do you feel about being vulnerable in front of/with your partner? Can you use the exercise above to create an opportunity to explore feelings about the birth?

Write a paragraph as if you are the empowered woman on the other side of giving birth. How do you feel? What do you look like? How will you take this experience into other areas of your life?

💡 SUGGESTIONS

Arrange a time to do the Feeling the Feels (Box 16) activity. If there is a lot of anxiety on either side about the birth or conflict about how to proceed, it can be invaluable to have someone else create a safe space to be able to hear each other.

If it's not something that your partner is comfortable doing, find a listening partner (Box 10) or a good friend or family member that you can share your feelings with.

Write in a journal or in the Reflections booklet you can download from www.pearlsofbirthwisdom.com/downloads.

🔍 RESOURCES

Brené Brown (2015) *Daring Greatly: How the Courage to Be Vulnerable Transforms the Way We Live, Love, Parent and Lead.* Penguin Life.

Jennifer Gunsaullus (2019) *From Madness to Mindfulness: Reinventing Sex for Women.* Cleis Press. (This has many helpful concepts and techniques that are just as relevant to birth as sex.)

Pearl 10
Trust

*Trust can carry you through
the unknown when you have
nothing else left.*

Imagine your newborn lying contentedly in your arms. This child is dependent on you for everything: food, shelter and love. Your baby is too small to know what trust is, but this will develop as you keep showing up for them. Every time you pick them up and wipe their tears away, their trust will grow. Each time you contain their anger or frustration, they'll know that they can count on you while they learn to navigate their emotions.

Not all of you reading this will have religious faith or spiritual connection that supports trust through a belief in a higher good, but through mindfulness and reflection, my hope is that you learn to trust your own inner strength and your amazing female body. Rather than expecting the health professional to guide you from start to finish, you can be guided from your previous life experiences and what you have learnt from them, from your body growing this baby so beautifully and from your current intuition of what is right for you.

Trust is a choice that you make, it cannot be demanded. Trusting others starts with trusting yourself and your body. Trust is a feeling of confidence and security, and this may seem difficult to create for a first birth, or where a first birth didn't go as expected when preparing for a subsequent one. However, the more situations in which you do trust your body, the more likely you can extend that to an unknown situation. We return to that need for feeling safe that is the central message of this book. Likewise, for your ability to be calm: the more situations in which you can keep your calm and know which techniques work to help you feel safe, the more you are able to trust that the same will be true in birth. This is why the preparation you make for the birth and all the techniques you learn will benefit many other areas of your life.

Next, we have a mother who shares her complete trust in her body and nature's way.

KELLY'S BIRTHING STORIES

(homebirths, no intervention)

Kelly runs a busy chiropractic clinic and is a champion for healthy living. She's a deep thinker and challenges herself to try new experiences all the time.

We have three children. On the surface the pregnancies and births all look similar but when Tessa asked me to put pen to paper it occurred to me how different they all were; rather let me clarify that with, how different I was!

Our eldest child is almost 12 and when I knew I was pregnant, I was super excited, shocked by how quickly it happened and acutely aware that I didn't really know what I 'should' do. I didn't have a GP, for reasons not super relevant to our birth stories but as we choose to approach health fairly differently from mainstream I had never registered, knowing if I ever needed a doctor it would be in an emergency and so I would go to A and E.

After asking a group of people I knew who had either had children or were pregnant, I realised that in order to have an appointment with a midwife, I first had to join a GP surgery. I booked my new patient appointment with a local GP, met with them, got told a basic 'due date' (that was actually calculated initially as three months later than I expected...that's a long pregnancy!) and given the contact details of a midwife I had to contact. This was all done in north London where we were living at the time. We were about to move to Berkshire, but I assumed (incorrectly as I later came to realise) that maternity care was similar across the board regardless of where you lived.

Professionally I had had a lot of interaction with midwives, health visitors and some obstetricians when I worked in Newcastle. So, I felt quite confident I knew what to expect. As it turned out it was entirely different in London and totally different being the 'patient' myself.

We met with a lovely midwife who came to the house where we were living at the time and she was very kind, asked a lot of detailed questions, and that's where my 'decision' was made. This very well meaning, and very enthusiastic midwife was approaching this pregnancy from an angle I wasn't prepared to embrace and really didn't like.

I knew I would have my children at home and she was keen to support us with this (indeed she was currently working towards becoming an independent midwife) BUT all her questions came from 'what if this is wrong, we need to check this is OK'. The whole appointment made me feel stressed and as if I wasn't in control of any choices. It was fear based as opposed to informative and it was in direct contrast to how we choose to live our lives.

I had previously, and extensively, investigated all the tests I would be recommended (blood tests, scans, growth checks, standard health checks like BP, urinalysis, etc.). I had read in detail (and had several years of familiarity of these tests from my own clients I care for) what they were testing for, how the tests worked and then what would be recommended if the test was positive. I feel information is key to anyone who is pregnant or wishes to become so, as only when you do your own impartial reading with a logical and non-emotional attachment to the information can you really start to make informed choices.

After the midwife left that day, I immediately said to my husband that we wouldn't be able to use the NHS and would need to find us someone else who was experienced and knowledge-

able and could support us with this pregnancy and birth. I didn't know where that would take us, but I did know of a colleague who had had her baby at home and contacted her.

She introduced us to an independent midwife and our journey took a totally different turn. Our midwife lived close to where our new home would be and after our booking appointment with her, we made the decision to work with her. She also asked a lot of questions, was very kind but the conversations where in stark contrast. Speaking to her was enlightening. She saw birth as normal and had a great deal of experience with births in general. Her background was as a trauma nurse among other medical areas and brought a great deal of experience in those areas with her. The main difference was that she expected things to go well and could quickly and easily offer us other suggestions when I told her we did not want to have the huge catalogue of tests recommended. To clarify I feel that those tests can be and are absolutely appropriate in some situations but not for the majority of women. For all three of our pregnancies I have had no monitoring, scans, blood tests or any other intervention. I did not check my urine, blood pressure or use a sonic aid to listen to the baby (during the pregnancy or birth), I also had no internal examinations. We have experienced two miscarriages, and despite this being very sad and distressing, we also decided to let those happen naturally. I am confident in my health and I know my body knows what to do. I of course monitor myself and sit quietly and see how things are but do not find it necessary or needed to ask for something external to reassure me that all is well.

We moved to Berkshire and shortly after that move our first child was born. It all started seven days before 'expected'. My waters broke at 2.30 Tuesday morning. I didn't have any discomfort, contractions or any other symptoms. I called the midwife and she reassured me to go back to bed, keep comfy and get as much rest as I could. After two days of doing that and bouncing on my ball things did start to ramp up. I had discovered that by bouncing on my ball I could 'control' the contractions and that was very nice!! Not so nice for getting on with having a baby. In hindsight I realise that the fear of the unknown was stopping me from embracing it and the concern over impending parenthood was actually quite overwhelming. So 'stopping' that was unconsciously what I was doing! I went shopping to Tesco's, pottered around and then decided to go for a long walk. I asked my husband to drop me around the corner and I would walk home; I had heard walking really got things ramped up. Sadly, what I hadn't realised was that being new to the area I didn't really know where I was, and my husband was right to be reluctant to drop me anywhere! About two hours later I finally made my way home and the walk had done a good job! My husband was still encouraging me to walk and move but I had found my faithful birthing ball and duly started bouncing away on it.

By Thursday lunchtime things weren't really changing. The midwife had been to us a few times and we kept her updated every hour or so on the phone. I suggested my husband go to work that morning, as there was no point staying at home if nothing was happening. My best friend who had been over for several hours for the past two nights had gone home and I also suggested she not come Thursday night as things were slow.

Well that was it. Being on my own with solitary focus, things went from about 0–60 in a few hours. My husband came home and we called our midwife who came in about 40 minutes.

I remember going to the toilet and having the best poo and biggest wee and just after that, transition happened and I got into the pool. I vomited (which I didn't enjoy obviously) and then felt much calmer and clearer. The mayhem of getting the pool filled quickly escaped me (as did the heat in the room) and I was oblivious of everyone else feeling hot and bothered! We had chosen to have no monitoring during the birth, so no heartbeat was listened to, I had no internal examinations and was left to *birth in the way I felt best. Our midwife listened to the noises and watched closely but from afar, careful to not interrupt.*

Just before his head was born, I clearly remember thinking I was going to die! Thinking it was not possible that women had done this for thousands of years and that the burning pain was too much. I cannot remember that pain at all now and didn't as soon as he was born. He was born into the water and did not cry and scream – just made a single 'squark' after a few minutes. My husband had spoken to my best friend and said if she wanted to be at the birth then she needed to come asap! She arrived during the birth and she was probably in the room for about 30 minutes when he was born! Quite a surreal and magical experience to share with people!

From the start of his birth (when my waters broke) it took him almost three days to arrive. I am forever thankful to have had the opportunity that we did in not having to stick to someone's imposed time scales. His birth could have had a very different outcome had we not done a lot of reading and had a supportive birthing team who had a lot of common sense and experience to be able to nurture this process.

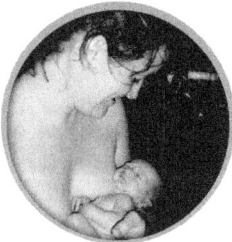

Fionn's Birth:

Our first child's placenta took 1.5 hours to be delivered, our second 45 mins and the third the placenta arrived within 15 minutes. It didn't occur to me to speed up this process and we did not opt to have any drugs to speed this up. This is also quite fortunate as all three placentas had a battle door insertion. This means that the umbilical cord goes into the side and not the centre of the placenta. In this situation if the cord is pulled to release the placenta (once artificial hormones have been given) the likelihood is it will snap. This then means the placenta must be surgically removed. Sadly, this situation is not as rare as some may think.

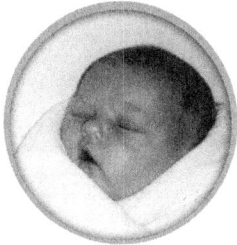

Faolan's Birth:

Our second birth we used our midwife again and he too was born in the same house as our first child, 18 months later. Again, he arrived almost a week 'early'. His pregnancy was the same in that we decided to opt out of all testing. His pregnancy was again without any challenges bar a significant bleed at 14 weeks. I spoke to our midwife and she reassured me. To this day we do not know if he was one of twins, but he was a great size, 8.4lb and came up with his hand and arm at the side of his head. I did not tear and had no injuries as a result. Not being rushed or stressed, my body was able to fully open up and birth him perfectly. The most stressful part of his birth was probably when our midwife said, 'if you would like to continue to slow thigs down you could lay down and rest'. He was coming quite quickly, and I had not realised that once again I was trying to control that. So instead I got into the pool and he was born within eight hours from start to end of his birth. Again, during his pregnancy and also birth, I was not examined and trusted my body knew what to do. Our midwife knew me well (continuity of care is vital for good birth outcomes I feel), had great experience to be able to listen and observe and know what was happening and where things were at. She was able to see things progressing well and able to be respectful to our choices and support a natural and empowering birth.

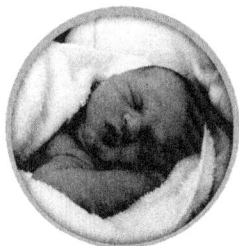

Ardan's Birth:

Our third birth was again at home, gentle and empowering. During the pregnancy once again, we had none of the suggested testing or checks. As it was six years later, it was different in what they were now recommending than when our first child was born. I found this interesting. I did the research again. Found out what the tests were, what they would do to do the tests (i.e. take blood), what they would do if the test was positive and what their recommendations would be. I wondered why some of the tests had changed dramatically since I was first pregnant and if anything, this made me even more confident to opt out of them.

We now lived in a different area and decided to look into someone more locally who would be able to support us. I am still to this day, delighted to have found our second midwife. She again was very knowledgeable and experienced but at a whole new level. She had supported hundreds of people who came from many backgrounds with very different beliefs and desires on how they wanted to have their birth play out. She had a wealth of research behind her (she loves information!) and was able to really, respectfully and safely support us. This time we also decided to look into hypnobirthing. A colleague had been teaching it and we had two private sessions with her. It is phenomenal and I have to say made a difference to the enjoyment of the birth. Our third child was born on 'the due date' (that we had calculated). His birth from start to finish was six hours and was awesome. I did once again hear myself saying, 'I cannot do this' and was amazed by the intensity of the birth but never once doubted it would all go smoothly and beautifully.

So, we have had three home water births, with two different midwives, on paper looking similar. They all felt very different and I believe that is led by the difference in personalities of the children now! It has been a great test of myself and my beliefs in my understanding of what my body can do. I trust my body knows what to do and with the right knowledge and support system it was nurtured and encouraged to do that. In the few cases where intervention is needed in birth it can be used and be super valuable. For the majority of births, I see a future where stories similar to those above are a reality for all women.

Kelly's story shows an incredible trust in the intelligence of the body and an acceptance of what will be will be. Knowing this mother personally, I know that her work as a body practitioner has led her to this point: it has been a journey. Such a hands-off approach will not be right for everyone, but often in the pregnancy class I see a shift from a desire for a medicalised birth to less med-icalised as women connect with their body's wisdom and birth as a natural process (see box). It's perfectly understandable to want reassurances in the forms of tests or the back up of being in the hospital and this book aims to reflect a whole spectrum of choices. What is most important is that each woman chooses the path that is right for her, and holds judgement when others do the same.

BOX 18: Trusting birth as a natural process visualisation

Take your awareness to your baby, safe and happy in your womb. Visualise or think about the umbilical cord that connects you together. Now imagine yourself as the baby, safe and happy in your mother's womb, linked by the umbilical cord and visualise or look at your bellybutton for evidence of the physical connection that once existed. Picture the umbilical cord that connected your mother to her mother, and your grandmother to her mother, and your great-grandmother to her mother, and back through the generations to your ancestors.

Birth has been happening for a long time and for most of history without intervention. Deep trust in birth as a natural phenomenon comes from knowing you are here today because all of these women before you that have given birth. We are so fortunate that today we also have medical support as another layer of safety. Repeat the affirmation silently three times: "My baby is safe. I am safe. A cocoon of safety surrounds us both."

ALICE'S BIRTHING STORIES

(premature, homebirth)

Alice is a gentle soul who I first met in a café. My youngest had gone over to say hello to the cute baby when she was just a few weeks old. Later Alice walked into my Mother and Baby Yoga class and we were trying to place where we knew each other from! Later she attended my Red Tent women's circle.

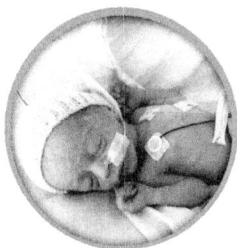

Flora's birth:

As soon as I got pregnant with my first child, I knew that I wanted the birth to be as natural as possible and we discussed a homebirth. I wanted to be totally present and feel the birth without any outside intervention. It was for this reason that we chose not to have the screening for Down's syndrome, we just wanted to trust in nature and the universe. However, when we went for our 20 week scan she was measuring small (on the 5th centile) but the consultant wasn't sure why or if it was a problem.

Being small is a risk factor for Down's syndrome and because we didn't have the test we were told to go back to the hospital for more scans. At each scan, the baby's growth continued to increase but she always measured on the 5th centile. We

219

were continually monitored and at 28 weeks I took steroids to help her lungs develop in case she had to be delivered early. Throughout all of this I had an overwhelming feeling that she was ok, and just naturally small.

We paid for a Down's syndrome test to be done privately which came back as 99.9% unlikely, and also paid for a private scan which showed that the blood flow supplying her was fine and she was indeed just small. However, at 34 weeks gestation we were told by the consultant that we would be induced because her belly hadn't grown since the last scan. I have used ultrasound equipment in my work before and know that measurements can differ through the day, let alone week by week. But of course, I did what they said because I'd never forgive myself if I went to full term and she wasn't ok.

We went up to the delivery suite to start the induction process, I had a pessary inserted for 48 hours because it was so early on in the pregnancy. She wasn't ready to come out just yet! Once the pessary was removed, I had to wait because the unit became very busy (apparently due to the full moon) and they didn't have time to start the induction properly. I was sent to have the drip inserted at one point but there wasn't a midwife available, so we were told to wait again.

During this time the baby was monitored every four hours and I was told she was fine. One of the midwives even mentioned she was a "Happy baby in there!". Eventually on day four (now 35 weeks gestation, yay!), the drip was inserted, and the induction began. I used some gas and air when the midwife attempted to break my waters, twice, with the doctor eventually managing to do it! However, I didn't get on with the gas and air, so I soon stopped using it.

I had been going to hypnobirthing classes throughout my pregnancy and I wanted the induction to have as little medical intervention as possible. Our midwife was wonderful and made the *hospital room as dark and peaceful as possible, and I had my relaxing music playing in the background. Charlie had a sleep on the floor, using his shoes as pillows, while I sat and breathed and listened to the music. I chatted with the midwife and felt fine!*

The surges started and I breathed through them, they weren't too painful to begin with but I was sick so the midwife offered me some anti-sickness tablets which I declined (I didn't want to start a slippery slope of medication). The surges started to get stronger and stronger and Charlie woke up from his sleep. I was able to breathe through each surge and our midwife said it was a very relaxed labour. However, towards the end of her shift the surges got extremely intense and I started shouting and making animal noises! The midwife asked the doctor if the drip could be turned down, but she said no. At the end of her shift the midwife checked how dilated I was - I was 2 centimetres so she swapped shifts with another midwife who said she would check me in a couple of hours. I remember thinking, I can't go on like this for another 2 hours!

Then the midwife told me to get on my hands and knees and I could feel a little hairy head travelling through my body. I didn't say anything though, I didn't feel like I was capable of speaking (although I felt very calm on the inside, as if I was just trusting my body. It was almost like an out of body experience). I was told the baby's heart rate was slowing down and that a monitor was going to be attached to the baby's head. When they tried, they realised that Flo was almost out!

And without any pushing (my body did it all on its own) Flora was born into the world at 0800hrs, weighing 3lb 4oz, exactly 12 hours after the induction began. Although my body and baby weren't ready (and despite one of the midwives telling me "You'll probably have a caesarean anyway because you're only at 34 weeks"), I calmly (for the most part!) delivered my baby without any pain relief.

After a very brief cuddle Flo was taken to the special care baby unit where she spent the first 12 days of her life. She was very healthy, absolutely no problems other than she needed to gain weight. I still believe that she would have been fine if she was left to spontaneously enter this world on her own, but I didn't have the confidence to say no to the induction. This all made my first experience of motherhood very difficult, but that's another story!

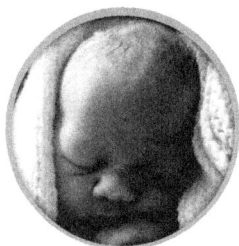

Wilbur's birth:

When I got pregnant again, I decided that if the same thing happened, I wasn't going to be induced, I would wait until labour started naturally. However, at the 20 week scan everything was fine and my baby was measuring on the 50th centile. Even so, we still had a couple of extra scans and initially we were under consultant care. One day I tentatively asked the midwife "Do you think I could have a home birth this time?" to which she replied "Of course! As long as your pregnancy remains low risk". So I was transferred from consultant care to the home-birth team!

I was so happy! Our midwife came to our house to do all of the midwife checks, which was wonderful. It was lovely to do all of the tests at home and for Flo to see too. We decided that Flo would be at home for the birth but that our neighbours would take her if needed. The rest of the pregnancy went smoothly, and I practiced hypnobirthing techniques every day along with reading lots of positive birth stories. Another thing that really helped me was doing visualisations every day. I visualised the baby in the best position for birth, head down etc, and I visualised the birth itself. From my waters breaking during the night in bed, to the moment Wilby's head could be seen - I imagined it all in positive detail!

At 3am on the 5th May (39 weeks gestation) I felt a 'twang' like a guitar string breaking. I thought, oh no what's happened?! Then a trickle of water came... my waters had broken! I felt very excited and quietly left the bedroom to tell my husband (Flo still sleeps in our room but Charlie was sleeping in the spare room at the time. He had had an accident on his bike a few weeks before and had fractured some bones so was sleeping upright in the spare room!). I told him my waters had broken but not to call the midwife just yet.

I went back to bed to be with Flo and the surges started. When they got a bit stronger I told Charlie to call the midwife and at about 4.30am she got to the house. I was still cuddling Flo in the bedroom as she wouldn't settle. I didn't go downstairs for a while but in the end the midwife said she'd really like to see me! So I went downstairs and the midwife asked me how the surges were feeling. They were stronger but I could handle them and speak through them so she said it was probably quite early on in the labour. She checked how dilated I was: 2cm again! She left to go home, as she had been at another birth all night and wanted to get some rest.

Charlie had already filled the birth pool. It was 42 degrees and we put a sheet over the top to keep it warm. Seeing as I could be labouring all day we didn't want the pool to cool down too much. The next two hours were wonderful: just the three of us and the dog. We diffused some essential oils, played my chosen music, and I sat in my 'nest' and did my relaxing hypnobirthing techniques. We had toast on the sofa and Flo would rub my back during the surges. She was the perfect birthing partner.

The surges were easy to manage, I would stop and breath

through them (doing the Golden Thread breath). I didn't find them uncomfortable and was expecting them to get much more painful. I was sitting on the sofa when I felt a transition occurring, I told Charlie I wanted to get into the pool but it was still too hot. He tried to cool it down and I started to feel the familiar feeling of a head transcending downwards! "I think the baby is coming" I said, and Charlie called the midwife but she was at home in bed. She told him to call an ambulance so he dialled 999. I told him I didn't want an ambulance, but he spoke to the emergency services anyway, answering lots of questions.

Meanwhile I had turned into a primal beast! Making the animal noises again which felt so good! But I was aware of Flo the entire time, who was sitting on the armchair opposite, taking everything in. I was still sitting on the sofa when the midwife burst through the door and told me to get on my hands and knees. I did, and she said "The heart rate is dropping". "Ah the baby must be coming" I remember thinking. This made me push, and Wilby was born into the world, onto the rug, next to the birth pool at 7.46am weighing 6lb 6oz.

I looked down and saw that he was a boy and I gave him his first hug. The paramedics had arrived and were sitting watching while Charlie, Flo and I all looked at this new little baby boy. After sitting on the toilet for a while to wait for the placenta, I decided to have the injection to expel it faster. If I had been in the birth pool I might have waited for it naturally, but at that point I felt like I wanted everyone to leave so it could just be us, my new family, at home together.

It was amazing having my baby at home, I would recommend it to everyone. My birth was quick and very relaxed, without much pain. I believe this was because I was at home, in a relaxed atmosphere, with people I trusted. Saying goodbye to the midwives when they left our home, compared to saying goodbye to my baby as I left her in hospital, was very healing for me. I believe everyone should have the chance to birth at *home, even if their [previous] pregnancy was 'high risk'. However, I will be forever grateful to the midwife in the hospital who made the room as relaxing as possible for me in the first labour.*

Like Kelly in the previous story, Alice had an innate trust in her body and the process of birth. Flora's birth story shows how challenging it can be to make decisions with the information you have. I love how she refocused for the second birth, using hypnobirthing techniques and positive stories to keep the trust strong.

DAVENE'S BIRTHING STORY

(sexual abuse trauma, episiotomy, homebirth)

Davene was not a yoga client of mine, but as the editor of the book felt moved to share her story of transformation and empowerment, and I am honoured to include it.

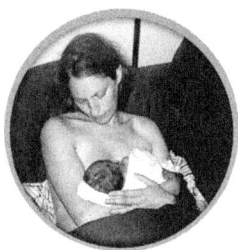

Elia's birth:

Years before I became pregnant, I watched a documentary with my husband called "The Business of Being Born." Once I learned how safe it was for a low-risk woman to give birth at home, I was sold. My husband wanted to look up the statistics that the movie referenced before he felt comfortable, but all the figures checked out, and he was very supportive of homebirth. When I was pregnant, I did everything imaginable to get my body ready: prenatal yoga, craniosacral therapy, massage, hypnobirthing classes – I went to birth conferences and even met Ina May Gaskin. (In the one-hour lecture she gave, she talked almost entirely about poop, which really put off a lot of the audience, but she was adamant that as women, we need to get comfortable with our bodily functions before we give birth, or else it's too hard to trust our bodies during labour.)

Two weeks before my due date, my mom, dad, and mother-in-

law rented a house within walking distance of me. (I was living in California, USA at the time, and our relatives were all on the other side of the country, near Washington, D.C.). It was a total nightmare. Every time I burped, one of the mothers would ask if I was in labour. I was constantly being watched, which did nothing for my ability to relax and trust my body and my baby. To make matters worse, my mother-in-law started hinting about wanting to be present at the birth. I had no intention of having any of my family at the birth – I was most comfortable with just me, my husband, and my two independent midwives. My mother in law wouldn't let up about wanting to witness the birth of her first grandchild. Finally, she told me that the moment I went into labour, she and my mom would start pacing up and down my street. "Don't be surprised if you see us peering in the blinds," she said, and I had finally had enough. I told her that if I saw her anywhere near my house while I was in labour, I would call the police. She finally got the message.

One day before I was 42 weeks along, I went into labour. Early labour was very long – 22 hours of dancing to my playlist, taking walks around the neighbourhood, and snacking on rice and beans (never eat beans during labour – worst idea of my life). The midwives came when I shifted to active labour, but it was still another 18 hours before my sweet baby would be born. The contractions were so strong – I didn't know then that my stomach was blown up like a balloon from eating all of those beans – the pains, mixed with the intensity of labour, was more than I could handle. I remember being in the birth pool and putting my head under water during contractions so the sensation of the water would give me a focus. I must have looked very strange!

At one point, I know my midwife was thinking about a hospital transfer. I have never been comfortable in medical settings. I find them very triggering, probably because I suffered from childhood sexual abuse. All I need is a white coat and a medical *instrument, and my body goes rigid. For that reason, I knew I would feel safest at home. But when labour had gone on for 36 hours, my body was so exhausted and the midwives were beginning to wonder if I could push through without medical help.*

I remember my midwife asking me, "How do you feel about how things are going?"

"Do you think I can have this baby safely at home?" I asked her.

"Yes, but you're going to have to work a lot harder," she told me.

I was so fearful of the hospital that I took her advice and really shifted into a higher gear. My other midwife told me to connect with whatever higher power I believed in, be it God, the Earth, my ancestors, anything. So I dug deep and I found strength I didn't know I had.

I remember the feeling of my baby moving past my pubic bone – she was right there! I was on the birthing stool and my midwife said, "This is one of the tightest fits I've ever seen. I have only cut one episiotomy in 20 years of practicing as a midwife. Do I have your permission to cut the second?"

When she asked this, I was in the middle of an intense contraction. I said, "Yes," not really knowing what else to say, because I hadn't counted on any intervention like this (and I wasn't really in the right mind to argue with anyone in the middle of a contraction). The sharpness and intensity of the pain felt so violent to me, I reared up off the birth stool and screamed. In that moment, I rejected my body, my pregnancy, all of my efforts to stay connected – I was in a rage – I was done and my anger gave me strength to push my baby out in the same contraction the episiotomy was cut during. Once she was born, the trauma from a moment before was replaced with the biggest surge of love and peace I have ever experienced in my life. My eyes were fixed on this perfect human that I had made. Elia was 8 lbs 15 oz.

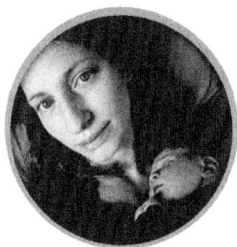

Sheina's birth:

When I became pregnant with Sheina, I lived on the east coast in Virginia, and initially found a midwife at a birthing centre who said she would come to my home and help me with a home birth. I told her about my sexual abuse, and asked that she please get my permission before she touched me at any point during the pregnancy or birth. She seemed very accommodating.

I began to feel uncomfortable at the next appointment, however, when she told me she was excited to be my midwife because, she said, "I never get to work with the 'cool' moms." I didn't know what that meant, but began to feel like she was seeking my approval in some way (NOT what I wanted in a midwife). Then she proceeded to do a vaginal exam without asking permission, and had completely forgotten about the traumatic episiotomy I had told her about at the first appointment. That was enough for me. Even though I had already paid $700 (homebirths are not covered by insurance in the US) and wasn't going to get any of the money back, I told her I was going to work with someone else, and then tried not to panic because I had no one else lined up and was entering my second trimester.

Within a few weeks, I found a wonderful midwife who had just moved to the area. She helped me process the trauma of my previous birth and encouraged me to do birth art to create a picture of what my first birth was like. I drew myself, and then cut out a section of the paper that went from my vagina up through my torso. The finished piece was essentially me, with a huge slice of my body taken from me.

The birth art I created illustrated my feelings powerfully – my memories of the last intervention were so violent (in large part because it had triggered my past abuse), and my midwife knew I would need to process those feelings to heal. I do want to point out that the episiotomy from Elia's birth was small (about 1.5 cm) and required no stitches. Still, it was very traumatic – both because of my past and because my midwife did not give me anaesthesia. I never thought to ask her why, and it makes me wonder if anaesthesia's something homebirth midwives typically carry with them in the US.

Because I had already given birth, I was not afraid of the pain. This time around, I spent less time reading every book I could find and filling my head with information, and more time connecting with my body and practicing mindfulness.

I remember one day when I climbed a ladder to my loft in the tiny country house we were renting, I banged my knee badly. Instead of cursing or freezing up, I just breathed through the feelings until they passed. This was my birth preparation. See what comes and breathe through without trying to get away or alter reality. When I went into labour – one day before my due date – I let the midwife and my sister know, and then went back to being in the zone. My sister started driving down (she was 2.5 hours north and was coming to be with Elia, who was now 4.5 years old).

I don't even remember when my midwife came. I was leaning into the birth ball, feeling the waves come and go, and I felt perfectly in tune with my body, with complete trust that it knew what to do to bring this baby into the world. What a feeling! Things progressed pretty quickly – a 7-hour labour in all – and when I felt the urge to push, I asked my midwife to check to be sure I was fully dilated. This was my request, not hers – I just needed the confirmation that it was time.

The pushing phase was actually pretty uncomfortable – I wasn't sure why, but something just felt off. At one point, I lifted one leg up while I was having a contraction on my knees (I was in the birthing pool at this point) and then I felt something shift and I felt much more comfortable. My midwife later told me that my baby's head wasn't positioned correctly, and that I had intuitively adjusted my body during a contraction to shift her position. I don't know how I knew to do that, but I knew! Sheina was born soon after.

I remember screaming for my four- year-old, because she was in the next room with her aunt and I knew she'd want to see her baby sister being born. Sheina's head was about to come out, and I realised I desperately needed someone to stabilize my perineum while I gave the final push. I just couldn't seem to find the words to ask someone to reach into the pool, so I reached down and caught my sweet baby myself! Never in a million years would I have dreamed that I could find the power to do what I did. I just reached down and pulled my baby up to my body like it was planned. I pulled her up to my chest and cuddled with her in the water a while before my midwife helped us into bed.

Sheina was 7lbs 15oz and perfectly healthy. My midwife was there the whole time to witness me, but aside from the one cervical check, and the occasional heartbeat monitor, I did everything myself. Sheina's birth is the single most powerful event of my life. I am forever grateful to her for helping me reclaim my own power – for helping me to become whole again.

The impact of sexual abuse trauma in labour and birth trauma is not talked about enough. Davene shows how powerful and empowering birth can be when we give ourselves the space and resources to process experiences and feelings. Midwives are not available in every state in the USA and sometimes travelling to another state is the only way to have that choice. In 2019, insurance was removed from Independent Midwives (working outside the NHS) in the UK and this left lots of women without the birth care that they knew would enable the level of trust with their health provider and their bodies. Thankfully, Independent Midwives are now able to work again.

It is critical that the birth partners also have trust in a woman's ability to birth. Both Kelly and Davene's partners understood their birth choices and how this would facilitate the best possible chance of the birth they desired. Sometimes in the birth preparation workshops, there are birth partners who have meditated, done mindfulness courses, or used hypnotherapy, and this always reassures me because they have repeated experience of how these states can benefit them. This is why I always include a relaxation during the workshop – mostly the couples will get comfortable on a couple of yoga mats and lie together spooning, both with a hand over their baby – because if the partners can experience how wonderful it feels to relax, they are more likely to support the mother during the birth to achieve this state.

Week after week in the pregnancy yoga, the women learn to trust that they can enter into this relaxed state and follow the cues of their bodies. If necessary, they listen to my voice on a recording talking them through a relaxation during the birthing journey, but often they have internalised it and no longer need an external guide. It is the repetition of listening and moving in the classes that works the magic and builds trust. I love Natalie Meddings' statement that 'birth remains a sum that doesn't add up'. There is something awesome about birth when you see it unfold naturally, and I still cry at every video of a birth that I see because there is something out of this world at play.

If you have realised through reading this book, that you experience a block to relaxing, feel a disconnection to your body or feel numb, I would suggest developing your 'felt sense' through Somatic Experiencing (see Peter Levine in Resources). The felt sense is bringing awareness inside your body (embodiment) to witness the ever-changing sensations, energies and emotions (see box). The felt sense moves us from a focus on what's happening outside in the world to qualities of our internal landscape. However, sometimes our natural ability to do this has been disrupted by a traumatic event. It may not be a big trauma; perhaps a bike accident as a child where you were not able to complete the stress cycle from having been scared and hurt.

BOX 19: Connecting with the felt sense

You might ask how is this different from mindfulness. Mindfulness is being aware of what is happening in the present moment without attachment of judgement. It creates space between ourselves and an experience. Experiencing the felt sense is about noticing a sensation in the body and not resisting it, but delving deeper to see what happens as you stay with it. The body often is a better record of our lives than our minds!

Get comfortable, either sitting or lying. Close your eyes and notice what sensations arise in your body. These might be sensations (like pressure, tension, pain, itching), temperature, shapes, weight, motion, speed, texture (like sandpaper, silk, stone, wood), absence/nothingness. (This is not an exhaustive list!). If it's hard to be with a negative sensation, you can move to a neutral or positive one.

If this is difficult, you can use a stimulus to help. Find something like a photo album or picture calendar (something where you won't be distracted by words). Look at the first picture and notice the sensations that arise in your body. Once you've named them, turn to the next picture and notice those sensations. Continue like this until you've felt different sensations in your body. (If this creates challenging feelings, you may wish to seek support from a Somatic Therapist or counsellor.)

Wild animals do not experience trauma according to Peter Levine, a psychologist specialising in trauma. When a rabbit has successfully tricked a predator by playing dead, it will come to and shake vigorously until the build-up of energy from the situation (preparing it for flight or fight) has been released. Humans often do not do this because the neocortex jumps in with thoughts like, "I'd better get up before anybody sees that I fell off my bike" and override the instinctive reaction to release energy. I've experienced both being able to follow my body's need to shake after being overwhelmed and overriding it.

The first situation was brought on by a feeling of utter helplessness on a cultural exchange trip at 13 years old where I blacked out. I was by myself and came to, shaking. I knew I had fainted from panic, but when the family I was staying with returned they insisted that I go to the hospital for a check-up. The second situation was a car accident where at first, I could not move out of my seat: not for any physical reason or for being trapped, but because my system had gone into freeze mode because I had no idea what had just happened. I did get out the car and soon ambulances arrived to take us to hospital for a check-up. However, I felt stuck in my numb state because the Doctor was very brusque in asking how I felt: I interpreted his attitude as judging that I had little to complain about when I had only whiplash when someone had died in another vehicle. For many years afterwards, I would involuntarily contract physically on motorways and feel adrenaline rising when another vehicle passed close by. It was only when I felt into the sensations and worked with my nervous system that this resolved.

Sometimes there is a reason why we do not innately trust our body, and I believe that often this is unresolved trauma of whatever scale. The beauty of Somatic Experiencing is that you do not have to go back through the event again and again, or even have to know what the trauma was, to be able to restore the nervous system to functioning normally and feeling safe in your body again. This is a wonderful way to move into motherhood.

REFLECTIONS on Trust

To have trust that things will happen the way they need to is a wonderful gift. In the same way that you will mother the child growing inside you now so that they trust you implicitly, you can mother yourself and trust that you will rise to the demands of this rite of passage. For my daughters I am always anticipating what they need for a journey: what food will they need, will they be warm enough, what will entertain them? You can prepare for your own needs in the same caring and thorough way.

Do you have religious or spiritual beliefs that can support you in trusting your safe journey through the birth of your child? What can support you to focus on these during the birthing journey?

What other experiences support you to trust the intelligence of your body and of the birth process? (E.g. tracking your cycle when trying to conceive made you realise the interplay of the hormones at play; attending yoga classes you found a new, positive relationship with your body; or reading positive birth stories helps you know what is possible for you.)

Write a list of all the times you've trusted your body or gut instinct (e.g. a foreboding about taking a certain path back home, or not wanting to eat something and it turns out it upsets someone else's stomach). Trust is built up from many tiny experiences that accumulate.

Do you essentially feel safe in your body? If not, do you know what has created this dis-ease? When you read or think about birth, what sensations arise in your body?

SUGGESTIONS

Regularly listen to relaxation or hypnobirthing tracks that contain affirmations about trusting your body and the process of birth. You can find a complimentary Yoga Nidra track at www.pearlsof-birthwisdom.com/downloads or visit www.yoganidranetwork.org.

Practice self-care every day.

RESOURCES

Peter Levine (1997) *Waking the Tiger: Healing Trauma*. North Atlantic Books.

Pearl 11

Everything changes

The only certainty is that everything changes.

In a moment I share two older birth stories to give you some historical context. Whereas a couple of generations ago, homebirth was the norm, the majority of women currently are birthing in hospitals. Many people since the 1940s have grown up believing that a hospital is the only place to safely have a baby. In my mother's generation, agency was handed in at the entrance to the maternity department door. You were given an enema and shaved as standard procedure. With my two birthing stories, you can see a change for the better!

In an ideal world, changes to care and to the policies that drive care are the result of high-quality research. You can search the National Institute for Clinical Health and Care Excellence (NICE) guidelines on many aspects of antenatal, birth and postnatal care to see what the evidence base is if you feel so inclined. The guidelines are based on the best quality evidence available, which would ideally be Randomised Controlled Trials (RCTs), but these have not always been conducted for a given topic and, in some cases, would be unethical to carry out. (It is unlikely you would get ethics approval to randomly assign women into receiving different levels of pain relief for example!) In private health care systems, which operate in much of the world, money and convenience also unfortunately drive how labour is managed.

Another relevant example of how public health messages have changed over time is how parents are guided to care for their babies. In the 1970s, parents were advised to lay babies on their fronts to sleep in case they vomited and choked. Currently the advice is for parents to lay babies on their backs. Weaning advice has also changed significantly over time, from when to start solids to what they can or cannot eat in the first year of life.

Currently, there are equal amounts of health promotion messages around encouraging breastfeeding and warning against co-sleeping with your baby. Given that ninety per cent of breastfeeding mothers will bring their baby into their bed at some point, this is unhelpful and confusing advice. (See Professor Ball's Infant Sleep research in the Resources.) Babies have not changed, but the thinking around babies keeps changing. This can feel like a minefield of confusing and often contradictory advice.

Having an overview of the context in which women give birth over time supports you to follow your intuition about what is right for you. We are incredibly fortunate that we have so much information at our fingertips because this was not available in the next three stories you will read. This knowledge lays the foundation for being able to decide what is right for you and your family. Preparing for the birth is a practice run for the myriad of decisions you will make for your child(ren) as they grow. Finding like-minded parents will support you in your choices.

Next, you'll read five birth stories connected to my family over different generations.

1950S:
AUNTIE EILEEN'S BIRTHING STORY
(homebirth)

Auntie Eileen is not my real auntie, but my mum's best friend. She still has a Cockney accent despite having left the East End of London decades ago.

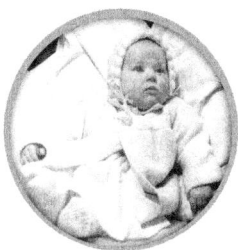

Lorraine's birth:

We lived in an old bomb-damaged Victorian house in Bermondsey, South London. It was really falling down. Two old men lived in the basement and we had three rooms on the first and top floor. There was no electricity and no bathroom; the toilet was at the bottom of the garden.

We were married for three months and I became pregnant. I had a trouble-free time once the morning sickness was past. The hospital said I would have a homebirth as I was young and fit. I didn't have a say in the decision they made. The hospital was Guys at London Bridge.

I worked up to two weeks before the big day. On 3rd November 1956, I developed really strong back pains, I could not sit or lie down. I just kept walking about. Charlie was watching TV and all he said was "Make us a cuppa". So much for romance!! I woke up on the 4th November at 5 o'clock with really strong pains, so I shoved Charlie out of bed and said "On yer bike, it's time, go get the midwife." He had to cycle to London Bridge to fetch help.

A very young man, he looked 15, turned up on his bike and set about giving me an enema. Nice! I had to struggle down three flights of stairs to get to the back garden to the toilet. It was a bitterly cold and foggy November day. I could not get off the loo, but somehow I managed to get back to the bedroom. How I did it I really don't know. I was holding my belly and my bum in case I had an accident.

The young man could not see what was going on, so he went downstairs to get the lamp off his bike. Charming! There I was in all my glory with this young man and a lamp peering at my nether regions! He kept shouting at me "Don't push, don't push". Well there was no one going to tell me what to do so I told him where to go. I was not a very good patient. Anyway, this went on for about 12 hours and finally my little bundle arrived at 6pm.

The young man called to Charlie for some newspaper. I thought "Surely he's not going to read!", but he put the afterbirth in the paper and gave it to Charlie and said, "Burn it." Good job we had an open fire. Lorraine weighed in at six and a half pounds. It really felt more like a baby elephant at the time. For the first four months I breastfed her and she was as good as gold, sleeping through the night every night, but then my milk dried up and she had to go on a bottle and she did not like that one bit. I never slept well after that for a very long time.

Enemas were a common practice to clear out poo (or 'manage potential leakage from the back passage' in euphemistic language), which tends to be squeezed out ahead of the baby's head descending. There's no danger to the baby in this happening during labour, and through the 1950s to the 1980s, it was still common practice to give a woman an enema for a number of reasons: it was thought to save the embarrassment of the mother, shorten labour, and give the baby more space. However, a Cochrane review (the gold standard of evidence-based medicine) in 2013 found that there were no benefits for the mother or baby.

All mammals (even herbivores) consume their own placenta, because it is nutrient dense and supports postnatal recovery. In many traditional non-Western cultures, the placenta is also eaten for this reason. Placenta encapsulation is the process of creating vitamin capsules out of the dried organ. This practice extends the benefits of the nutrient-rich placenta, but in a form that is easier to take. Some of my clients have used this service and shared that they felt that it protected against post-partum depression. I don't know of any research studies on the effects of placenta ingestion, but there is lots of anecdotal support for it, including the editor of this book who shared her personal experience with me:

Davene said,

> *My mother had severe postpartum depression after birthing my older sister. Her depression after my birth was even worse, and kick started a decade-long clinical depression. Her mother (my grandmother) was even worse – after her first child was born, she had postpartum psychosis and checked herself into a mental health ward. This was the 1950s – and the thinking on mental illness (in the US anyway) was very backwards. My grandmother got electric shock treatment at the facility and was very traumatized. Hearing these stories growing up, and knowing how sensitive the women in my family are to hormonal fluctuations, I was determined to do everything I could to not follow in their footsteps. I researched how to prevent post-partum depression, and decided to encapsulate my placentas from*

both births. I am happy to report that I did not suffer from post-partum depression, and feel strongly that the nutrients and hormones from the placenta played a major factor in this, helping to ease my body off the pregnancy hormones, instead of dropping off the hormonal cliff.

1950S:
ROS'S BIRTHING STORY

(homebirth)

Kathi is my mum and is a down-to-earth type of woman and her mother was much the same. In Yorkshire, you call a spade, a spade and just get on with things!   My grandmother Rosalind is sadly no longer alive, but my mum recounts what she knows about her birth.

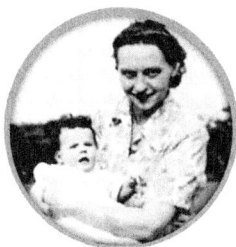

Kathi's birth:

I was born on 10th March 1950 in Barnsley. My two sisters were born pre-NHS in nursing homes. I don't know whether cost was involved in the decision to have a homebirth, but my parents would have had to pay doctors, nurses and medicine fees for their first two children. It's possible that a homebirth was covered by the NHS whilst nursing homes may still have been private.

On the day of my birth, the midwife called to examine my mother, who was told that there was quite a time to go and she would be back later in the day. Shortly after, my mum called my father to say the baby was on its way and could he go and fetch the doctor.

There was no telephone in those days, so after leaving my mum in the not-so-capable hands of a neighbour, he ran to the doctor (who tended to us throughout our childhood). The neighbour was panicking so mum sent her out of the room and proceeded to deliver me on her own. The story always stopped here, and I know nothing else about the birth!

I loved hearing about the continuity of care from the same doctor from birth throughout my mum's childhood. They lived in a small two-up, two-down terraced house without a bathroom at the time she was born, and I can still picture the kitchen where it all happened.

1970S:
KATHI'S BIRTHING STORY

(hospital birth, ventouse)

My dad worked abroad for a while and was delighted to have the experience of travelling to different parts of the world. We lived in Kenya for a few years before moving to Malawi and so I was born abroad. Here is the story of my birth.

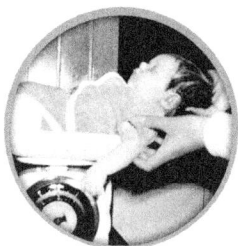

Tessa's birth:

Tessa was born in Nairobi, Kenya. All medical services were private, so I went to see a gynaecologist (in a tower block – thank heaven for lifts) from South Africa. I was booked into the main Nairobi Hospital for a week, payable in advance. I was really well throughout my pregnancy – no sickness. I did put on rather a lot of weight and it was decided when I was two weeks late that I should be induced.

I was told to arrive on Sunday afternoon, ready to be induced on the Monday morning. I was given an enema and shaved. Within a few hours I began labour. I remember complaining to her dad that my back was really aching and blaming the uncomfortable bed. No walking around – it was, "get in bed and stay there". It never entered my head to say, "I'd much rather walk around".

Every so often someone popped their head around the door and checked me, but dad-to-be was sent home to get some rest as there was "No point in him hanging around" and I felt really alone. Eventually it was decided that it was time to call the consultant, which was not my lovely Mr P., but another one who was covering weekends. My gynaecologist was away for the weekend and would not be arriving until 9am.

Tessa decided she couldn't wait and I was taken to the delivery room. Her dad arrived and she was born shortly afterwards. I do recall that I didn't much like the lady doctor. She was rather brusque and just getting on with it. After a discussion with nursing staff, who left the room, returning with a trolley, she took some equipment from it. I remember thinking "The baby's dead and they're taking it away". She didn't explain what was happening, but of course I know now that it was the vacuum extractor [ventouse]. I was told that the decision was made because I was tiring and Tessa wasn't moving down the birth canal.

I often think now that had I been encouraged to walk around and not had to lay down, gravity might have helped! I had stitches, but only a few. I was advised to have salt baths.

Tessa was 7 lb 4 oz with lots of hair.

My mum always talked very positively about being pregnant and having her babies. However, when I read the story that she'd handwritten for me in a letter, I thought of all the big, negative emotions that she felt due to the way the labour was handled.

I do tend to rush through life because there's so many wonderful things to see and do, and I wonder whether this propensity comes from the ventouse pulling me out before I was really ready! I'm sure Anna Verwaal [mentioned in Pearl 2], the Dutch Maternal-Child Health Nurse, would have lots to say about that.

2010S:
MY BIRTHING STORIES
(hospital transfer, waterbirth, homebirth)

As you know from the introduction, I had been doing meditation and yoga for many years before starting a family. I had trained to teach pregnancy yoga the year after completing my general yoga training and loved it from the beginning. I only learnt to teach mother and baby yoga after having my own children. I started antenatal care in Bristol, but transferred to Reading at eight months pregnant. I worked as an academic researcher at the Bristol Royal Infirmary until the maternity leave of my second child.

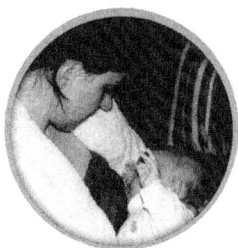

Zara's birth:

I went into the hospital for the booked induction at 42 weeks pregnant, knowing that I was going to decline the intervention if the baby seemed happy. I had always thought that the due date was too early and we have a history of having overdue babies in my family. The monitors reported that everything was fine and the midwife talked about giving me a pessary to start the induction. I declined the pessary and agreed to active management: that I would come in every day to have the baby's heart rate and blood pressure monitored.

The midwife was called away because they were very busy that day and when she returned, she said that she would get the pessary and I could go home. I reminded her that I had declined the pessary and she suggested a sweep. She was then called away again and when she returned, she apologised about the delay and would sort out the pessary! I think it was just that this would be standard procedure and so she was defaulting to this course of action. In her absence I had decided to have a sweep and so she went ahead with this; it felt fine, not uncomfortable at all, which I believe indicated that my body was getting ready for labour anyway.

We went home with the promise to return tomorrow for more monitoring. In the afternoon I pottered around the house and went to bed around 9pm, leaving my husband in the lounge writing on the computer. The birthing pool was inflated in that room and I was planning a homebirth. After midnight I woke up with what felt like period pains, except that they were coming and going. I got up and went downstairs to find my husband Fabio still on the computer. He couldn't believe that these were contractions when he hadn't had any sleep yet!! (As an aside, Fabio is from Italy and birth is more medicalised there. He quickly came on board with a homebirth, but we didn't tell his family about our homebirth plans until after the event.)

I sat on the birthing ball for a while and since the contractions were already coming regularly, I asked him to time them. I also spent some time lying on my side on the sofa, listening to a hypnobirthing track in a dreamy state. As the contractions got closer together, I couldn't wait to get into the pool, and asked him to start filling it as I thought I'd be most comfortable there. Within 20 minutes it was at the minimum level and I eagerly got in, feeling instant support and relaxation.

Once the surges were coming every three minutes, Fabio rang the triage line and the midwife spoke to him, and then she asked to speak to me. Classically I was in the middle of a contraction and had to wait to speak to her. I handed the phone back to

Fabio as another one started and he explained that we were planning a homebirth. Unfortunately, the midwife said that there wasn't someone to come out. There wasn't a dedicated homebirth service in the area at the time and I didn't realise that it was a possibility that there was no midwife to attend.

It was a real shock. I had just not imagined that a resource issue would prevent me from having a homebirth: that hadn't been mentioned at all as a possibility. I knew that I could say that I wasn't going to move, and they would have to find someone, but both Fabio and I didn't want to do that. According to the midwife on the phone, the (only) birthing pool was currently available and there was a chance that I would be able to use it if I came in now.

We decided to head into the hospital. One of the most difficult parts of the birthing journey for me emotionally was getting out of the birthing pool where I was so comfortable and getting dressed in between contractions. The car journey was also the most intense part of the labour because I couldn't move as freely. I was so relieved to arrive at the maternity department and get out of the car.

When I arrived, I was immediately examined, and the midwife was surprised to find that I was 6cm dilated because I was so calm. We had a bit of a wait in the assessment room and I remember feeling a bit despondent because it was so clinical compared to my lovely familiar and cosy lounge at home where I'd planned to birth. However, once we got into the room on the delivery suite it was much more relaxing because it had been made to look like a bedroom, with a double bed, bedside tables with lamps, a birthing ball and armchairs (covered in easy clean material!). I wasn't in there very long before I moved next door into a different room with a birthing pool and Roman mural on the wall. Such bliss to get back into the water.

A few times the midwife asked me to get out of the pool to go to the toilet and be examined, and each time I was very re-

luctant. I had a vest on, but felt uninhibited, even about the little bit of poo that would sometimes appear in the pool. The midwife was lovely and unobtrusive. She was constantly measuring the temperature of the pool water and writing notes: she was in the room, but in the background and letting me get on with it. I moved around in the pool, spending some time leaning forwards, and other times, resting my back on the edge of the pool. I used some gas and air towards the end, and Fabio also tried it when the midwife wasn't looking. I don't remember it particularly making a difference, but I was holding on to the mouthpiece like a safety blanket.

As I started to feel that I wanted to push, the midwife asked me to get out of the pool to check that I was fully dilated. Urgh I really did not want to do that. Fortunately, it didn't take long and I got the go ahead to push. I got back in the pool and it was an overwhelming urge to push that came from my body rather than my brain. I focused on breathing long and slow, and resting after a contraction was finished. I remember the burning sensation of the perineum being stretched and it really helped to reach down and feel the baby's head right there.

Fabio was videoing this bit, but I was oblivious to it at the time. I don't remember the second midwife coming into the room at all. My total focus was on the sensation of the baby's head being right there in my vagina. Incredible! I also remember waiting with her head out of me, waiting for the next contraction to birth her shoulders. Then suddenly the midwife was guiding her up through the water and up to my chest. Then I was crying and laughing and feeling a rush of love. It was the first time I had ever seen my husband cry. It was an overwhelming moment and I felt euphoric.

Beforehand, Fabio had not wanted to cut the umbilical cord. However, in the moment, he could not wait to get involved and cut the cord once it had turned white, while I was still in the pool.

251

After a cuddle and cupping water over my baby to keep her warm, the midwife suggested I get out of the pool to deliver the placenta. It was so hard to get out of the lovely warm water. I had a towel around the baby and I and sat on the birthing stool. I have no recollection of how long the placenta took to come, but Fabio reckons it was about 30 minutes. I coughed a few times and felt it slither out on to the pad below. The baby was weighed and checked over, and Fabio never took his eyes off her in case she got mixed up with someone else's baby!

After that we moved back to the bedroom-like room next door and on route my daughter emptied all the meconium poo out in one go down my pyjama trousers. These had to be thrown away along with a pillowcase that had somehow got covered too! We snuggled into the bed and started our breastfeeding journey. She latched on beautifully and stayed there for about an hour.

Then I needed to move to another room to have stitches for a second-degree tear and the midwife said she would bring a wheelchair. I protested, saying I felt fine, but she insisted that since I had just had a baby it might be nicer. And so I said good-bye to the wonderful midwife Dorothy, who I shall never forget for delivering my first child.

A different midwife came to do the stitches and I found the gas and air much more useful then. At one point I farted in the mid-wife's face and she did an admirable job of not looking disgust-ed. My excuse is that the local anaesthetic meant I had no con-trol over my pelvic floor at all. Halfway through, the supervisor of midwives came in to ask the stitching midwife a question about something (not to do with my care) and I felt it was weird that she did not introduce herself or acknowledge me in any way given that I was lying there with my legs open in stirrups, but was too tired to say anything.

Fabio at the time was holding our baby very tenderly. Once the stitches were done, I had a shower on now wobbly legs (I think the adrenaline had worn off) and then climbed into bed to have another cuddle with my baby. Finally, the tea and toast arrived, and nothing had ever tasted so good.

Once the consultant had come in to check her hips and another observation had been done, I was told I could get her dressed and take her home that evening as I'd been planning a home-birth and didn't want to stay in hospital. I hadn't expected her to be 8 lb 11, so had only one baby outfit that was big enough for her and had to borrow an NHS blanket to keep her warm. It was wonderful to get back home to pizza on the sofa and my own bed.

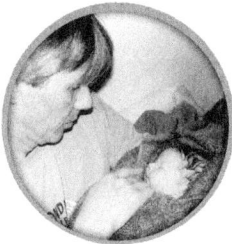

Alma's birth:

When I was planning the second baby's birth two and a half years after the first one, I was determined to have a home-birth, so I employed an independent midwife (the dedicated homebirth team was not yet set up). I was extremely fortunate that my husband's health insurance covered this, but other-wise would have considered a doula who could be my advo-cate. One of the benefits of an independent midwife is that you consistently see her through your pregnancy and have longer appointments, averaging about 45 minutes. This gives her an opportunity to get to know you.

I was determined to finish painting the hallway and cloakroom before the baby arrived. So until 3pm on the day that I went into labour I was up a ladder with an Apple Green paint pot and my mother looked after the toddler. I then felt tired and so lay down on the sofa for a rest. When my husband came back from work at 6.30pm I was still there and wondering whether the contractions had started. This was 41 weeks + 1 day. Fabio put pizza in the oven, and I ate this still lying on my left side on the sofa.

At 9pm, Fabio called the midwife to say that I was having regular contractions. She talked with me between contractions and said it would be best to have some sleep and to ring her again if this sped up. I went upstairs to have a bath because there was no way I could get to sleep. I couldn't get comfortable on my side or back in the bath, so was leaning forwards against the end wall during contractions and going into a wide-legged child's pose in the expansion phase. Meanwhile I'd asked Fabio to fill the birthing pool in a downstairs room, but it was taking ages and he had two kettles on the go, with my mum scuttling backwards and forwards with hot water (having put my eldest to bed previously).

Going back to the labour... Fabio had lit candles in the room downstairs to make it cosy, but I was upstairs alone in the bathroom waiting for the pool to be warm enough. I was very happy there by myself, focused on my breathing. Every time a contraction came I imagined a wave washing up my legs into the cave of my womb and gently drawing the baby down. I must have imagined that hundreds and hundreds of times, but it helped the most in travelling through the intensity of the contractions. I had to ask for extra towels for under my knees because the bath was really hard.

At some point, an hour after the first phone call perhaps, Fabio had called Amber again saying that the contractions were getting closer and she said she was setting off from home 45 minutes away. When she arrived, she brought her kit inside and came up to the bathroom. As she walked in, I said, "I feel like I want to push" and she said, "Go ahead". It was so differ-

ent from my first labour with multiple examinations. I stayed kneeling in the bath, pushing against the end wall during the contractions. Very soon afterwards, I could feel her head moving down into my vagina and I shouted to Fabio to come as the baby was arriving. He rushed upstairs (from the pool which he was still trying to fill!) and came in just as she was born. I remember the midwife saying, "You're amazing Tessa" and I thought YES, I AM!!

I had felt in two minds about having my mum in the house when I was in labour, but in the end, practicality won because I needed someone to be responsible for my daughter if she woke up. Although my mum and I are close and have been open about all sorts of things in my life, I wasn't sure if I'd feel inhibited and that would affect the course of the birthing journey. As it was, I called for my mum moments after the baby was born and lifted the baby in front of me, saying "Look the baby is here". She looked genuinely surprised as I had been quiet and she'd been focused on the pool downstairs, not realising how quickly the birth journey was progressing. At the same time, my older daughter woke up and so my mum went to her room. I sat on the toilet holding Alma, with a towel around us, and soon after, the placenta plopped out onto the mat that was across it. I have no memory whatsoever of Fabio cutting the cord, but apparently that is what happened.

The pool was now ready (a bit late haha!) so I decided that I wanted to get in and have a cuddle with Alma there. My mum brought Zara into the room to meet her new little sister and she said "Don't worry baby, Zara is here", which opened my heart wider. The midwife started to worry that we would get cold so we got out, were wrapped in new towels and she weighed the baby (8lb 12). I then fed her lying down, while Amber checked me for tears and found that there was a very slight one that didn't need stitches. I then took up camp in the lounge, back on the sofa where it had all started while the midwife tidied ev-

erything up. I started feeding Alma and soon afterwards Amber left, leaving us as a family of four and with a grandma with a different experience of childbirth!

By the late afternoon, my dad had arrived and just as we gathered in the lounge to have some champagne, the GP arrived to check us over. He seemed genuinely happy to have such a reason for a house call (but declined the champagne). It was amazing to be at home, to eat my own food and sleep in my own bed. It was reassuring to know that Amber the midwife would be back tomorrow to check how we were doing. Although it hadn't gone exactly how I had imagined it (using the pool after the birth, alone for most of the active labour in the bathroom), it was wonderful. I woke up the next day with a very tender forehead where I had been pressing it against the bathroom wall during contractions and bruised knees. The after pains were also much stronger this time, and where I hadn't had any pain relief during the birth, I needed paracetamol and ibuprofen. However, I felt like a heroine and that I could do anything.

In Italy, where my husband is from, obstetric care is the norm and midwives are not always available in every region. We decided not to tell his family about the plan for a homebirth until after the event as we thought they would worry. Reading other fathers' experiences of homebirth is what convinced him about the benefits of that choice.

In Reading, Berkshire, where I teach pregnancy yoga there is cultural diversity, perhaps due to the proximity to London. There are people from all over the world who come to the classes and share what the norm is for antenatal, birth and postnatal care back home. Many expectant mums from 'developed' countries, are surprised that they are not assigned an obstetrician or that there are not more scans and tests conducted. This can create a feeling of lack of safety if the reasons are not explained, which is that if a pregnancy is healthy and normal there is not the need for further intervention.

For parents who are not familiar with the local health care system, there can be extra barriers to creating this feeling of safety from language issues to a feeling of not being entitled. A lovely couple from the Lebanon became utterly confused and bewildered when the midwife talked about the need to move into the theatre. Theatre in their English lessons had only been used in relation to plays, never in a medical context. Some birth partners who are in the UK on a visa have admitted that they are scared to advocate for their partner in case this affects their ability to remain in the country. This stress is not fair or helpful during the birth journey and I would encourage the couple to seek someone who feels confident to act as advocate for them.

Maternal outcomes for black and minority ethnic women are worse than for white women in the UK and getting worse. For example, black women have a higher mortality rate than white women in the perinatal period. Cultural safety and cultural humility are important if this is to change. Mars Lord, a birth activist, argues for black birthkeepers for black women. It is important to reflect on who would be the most empathic and able to advocate for you during the birth journey.

For some people, there isn't a baseline of safety. There may have been situation after situation that has traumatised them, like racism. As epigenetics has shown, trauma can affect us as a foetus in the womb and in our very DNA through what has happened to previous generations' bodies. But everything can change, and it is possible to release the trauma the body holds through modalities such as somatic therapy. Simple practices such as in Box 19 in the previous chapter can start the journey to creating what a sense of safety feels like. I thoroughly recommend Resmaa Menakem's book for a thorough, practical way forward.

In many cultures, women observe a period of seclusion after birth to recuperate. This may be as long as 40 days, in which time the mother is brought nourishing foods, kept warm and supported to rest. One Indian mother described how when she returned home to India to introduce her daughter to her family, the cleaner asked who had done the postnatal care for her in England. Who had massaged the baby? Who had massaged the mother? She was shocked that no-one had done this and said that even she, with a husband who was a night watchman, had afforded that service! We have much to learn from the postnatal culture of other traditions: supporting a babymoon to support establishing feeding and the mother's recovery. In Western cultures, there is an overwhelming message that we should get back to normal as soon as possible. This puts a huge burden on new mother's mental health, especially when they're expected to cope without wider support beyond their partner.

This brings us full circle back to soothing. When the baby is born, it is about soothing their nervous system in this strange new world that they find themselves in. Being in your arms is the place where they feel safe. Imagine how they go into flight, fight or freeze if they do not feel your protective arms around them. So begins a lifetime of their learning how to care for their own nervous system to enable them to travel through the rites of passage that await.

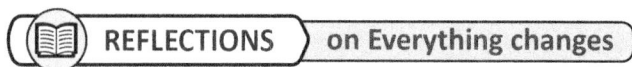

REFLECTIONS 〉 on Everything changes

Before choosing a question to reflect on, take a moment to imagine the time after your baby is born with the hard work done. This moment of gazing into your baby's eyes is something to hold onto tightly through the journey.

What do you know about your birth and the culture of birth at the time? When people talk about birth to you, are they talking from experience of a different time where practices were different?

Ask friends and colleagues from other countries about what the norm is for birth where they are from. Ask them to talk in generalisations unless they have a positive story to share.

Is it relevant to think about cultural safety in your birth preferences? Are there particular cultural practices that you want to be observed during your birth journey?

What are your plans for after the baby is born? What support can you ask for or arrange? Do you feel pushed to 'get back to normal' as soon as possible? What are your expectations in terms of how your day-to-day life will look, for your body, for how your baby will sleep or feed?

SUGGESTIONS

Write a postnatal plan for the first month post-birth to detail where your support will come from when the baby is born and explicitly what tasks you might like people to do when they come around. If you can afford it, perhaps consider a postnatal doula or a cleaner for a few months, or a supermarket delivery. Know that it is ok for your home to be messy.

Consider how you can make your baby feel safe in the first few hours after birth. You could stipulate that weighing and cleaning the baby can wait until after the first feed. Is there a necessity for your baby to be taken away from skin-to-skin contact where s/he can feel the warmth of your skin and familiar voice? How can you create the cocoon of safety for your baby that you felt during birth? Add these thoughts to your birth plan.

🔍 RESOURCES

Meredith F. Small (1998) *Our Babies, Ourselves: How Biology and Culture Shape the Way We Parent*. Anchor Books.

Heng Ou (2016) *The First Forty Days: The Essential Art of Nourishing the New Mother*. Tantar.

Kimberly Ann Johnson (2017) *The Fourth Trimester: A Postpartum Guide to Healing Your Body.* Random House.

Naomi Stadlen (2004) *What Mothers Do: Especially When It Looks like Nothing*. Piatkus books.

Deborah Jackson (2003) *Three in a Bed: The Benefits of Sleeping with Your Baby*. Bloomsbury Publishing.

Diane Wiessinger, La Leche League (2004) *The Womanly Art of Breastfeeding*. Penguin Group

https://abueladoulas.com/mars/black-maternal-health-week/

Resmaa Menakem (2017) *My Grandmother's Hands: Racialized Trauma and the Pathway to Mending Our Hearts and Bodies.* Central Recovery Press.

https://theblackdoula.com (Aims to bring equity to birthing people worldwide)

Juno magazine (Parenting magazine that focuses on attachment parent, natural living, etc.).

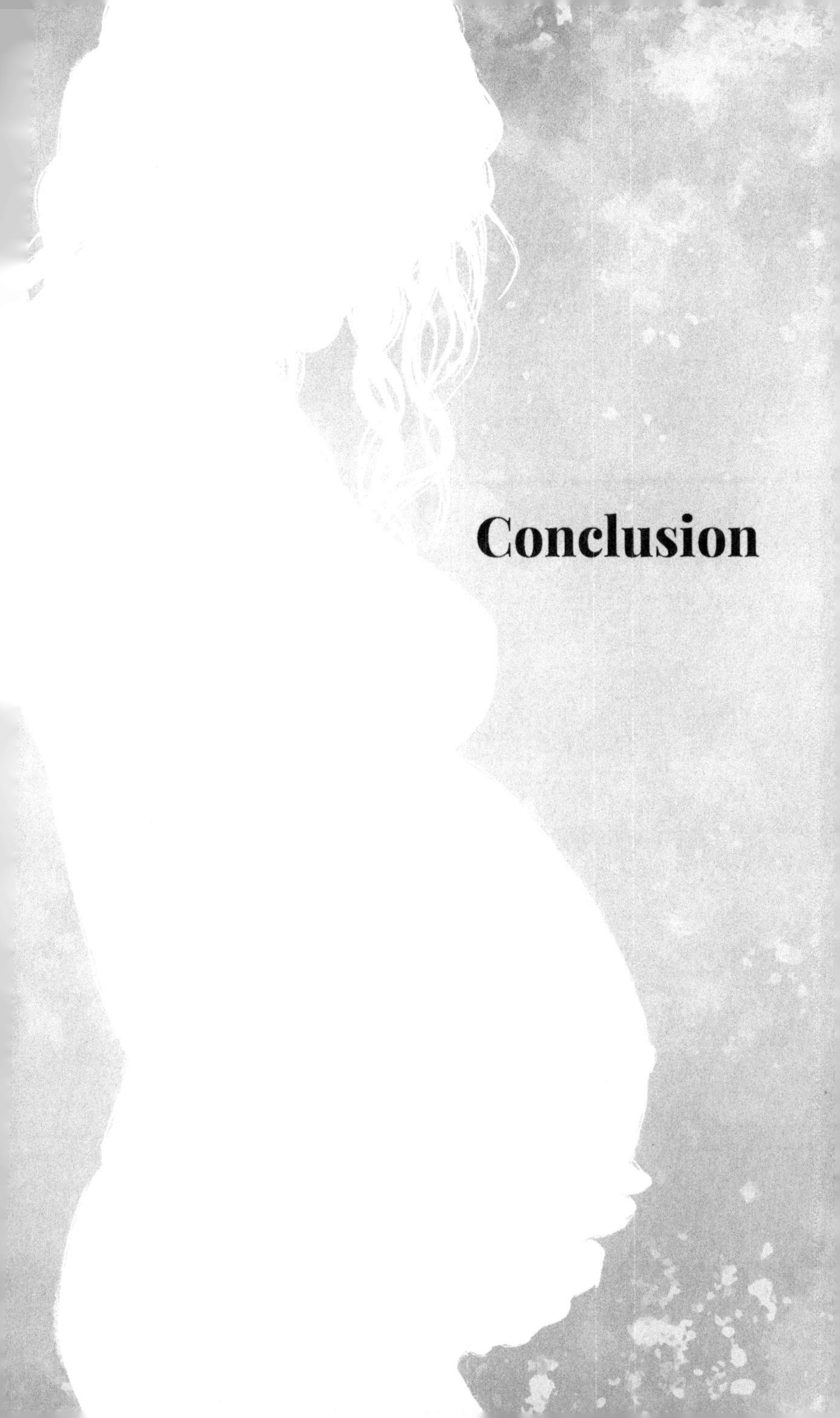

Conclusion

A vision for expectant mothers

My dream is that each woman will receive support from a consistent caregiver throughout her entire pregnancy journey.

My dream is that each woman will have access to knowledge that enables her to comprehend the magnitude of this rite of passage, prepare fully and feel empowered to make the decisions that are right for her situation, personality and body.

Every woman deserves to feel free to move during her labour and have birth professionals who trust women's ability to give birth, giving each unique mind-body space and time to find her way.

I want new mothers to feel supported to feed their babies and nourish themselves in the postnatal time, to safeguard physical and mental health.

My dream is that women have the choice of birth (e.g. natural, medicated, water, hypnobirth) and birth location that is right for them.

My dream is for all women in labour have the emotional support they need from loved ones or birth professionals like doulas, including those with previous trauma, single mums, young mums, mums pregnant with their first baby, mums pregnant with their fifth baby, mums in hospitals, in homes, in prison. Everyone!

A note on menstrual cycles

After the birth of your baby, the timing of the arrival of your first period will depend on whether you are breastfeeding or not. If you are bottle feeding, it is likely that your period will return after six to eight weeks. For mothers who are breastfeeding long-term, almost 50% are likely to restart menstruation between 12 and 24 months. Having travelled through the rite of passage of birth, this is an opportunity to develop a new relationship with your body and your menstrual cycle.

After the birth of my first child, I started tracking my cycle, not to maximise the chances of conception (I wasn't ready for that for a good while!), but to understand how my feelings and energy were affected through the whole month. I have noticed patterns of behaviour that enable me to be kinder to myself around the pre-menstrual phase, rest as much as is feasible with young children, and maximise productivity in the ovulatory phase. This knowledge supports me to pace and balance work and family activities, and care for my nervous system. Self-care is prioritised because I know this helps me to be the mother that I want to be for my children.

New mums can easily take on the lion's share of childcare and not have time for self-care. This might affect the pre-menstrual phase when menstruation returns, sometimes resulting in a rage like never experienced before. Sometimes, I have mums who message me, worried about their mental health and wondering what is happening to them. If they can ask for the support that they need from their partner, family or friends, the rage recedes, and balance is regained. Tracking your cycle when it returns can give you peace of mind.

You may also rethink the menstrual products that you use, perhaps trying organic products that do not put chemicals in contact with your vulva or vagina, menstrual cups or reusable pads. These steps can often reduce heavy flow and increase awareness of how flow changes over the days of the bleed.

Where women have practiced cycle awareness before pregnancy, often there is already a deep respect for the female body and the journey that we have undertaken is already underway. My hope is that many more women in the future will experience their cyclical wisdom and this will lead to trusting the journey of pregnancy and birth more easily.

(Q) RESOURCES

There are a growing number of books about how to practice cycle awareness and the benefits that this can bring, and how to support healthy periods. Here are my favourites:

Alexandra Pope and Sjanie Hugo-Wurlitzer (2017) *Wild Power: Discover the Magic of Your Menstrual Cycle and Awaken the Feminine Path to Power.* Hay House.

Toni Weschler (2003) *Taking Charge of Your Fertility*. Vermillion.

Lara Briden (2017) *Period Repair Manual*. Createspace.

Natasha Richardson (2020) *Your Period Handbook: Natural Solutions for Stress Free Menstruation*. Aeon Books.

Stacy Sims (2016) *Roar: How to Match Your Food and Fitness to Your Female Physiology for Optimum Performance, Great Health and a Strong, Lean Body for Life.* Rodale. (Aimed at athletes but an incredible wealth of information about diet and exercising for anyone with a menstrual cycle.)

Clue App – If you prefer Apps to pen and paper, this 'period' App is the one most used by girls and women who attend my workshops. Others exist with different options and functionality so see what suits you.

A note on menopause

The major rites of passage in a woman's life are menarche (first period), birth, menopause and death. In some traditional societies, there are special practices or information given to girls as they start menstruating. The elder women or the whole village provide a safe container as the girls mature into their sexuality. Pregnancy and birth provide another life experience that deepen women's understanding of what they are capable of, if supported well. A difficult onset of periods can cause a challenge when it comes to preparing for birth: there might be issues to resolve around the female body, such as shame or distrust.

I strongly believe that if these opportunities for inner work are not taken and supported at the time of the rite of passage, they reappear during menopause. In our society, we mainly focus on the physical symptoms of hot flushes, night sweats, fat gain around the middle, memory issues and mood swings. Officially entering the menopause is not having had a period for one year. However, there is a psycho-spiritual journey that happens within this ten-year phase to mature us into wise women, that may or may not coincide with the physical symptoms.

A friend of mine cheerfully announced that she was post-menopausal, and I was surprised because she had described major physical symptoms from the hormonal changes, but no mental effects. I asked her whether she'd like to come to the Red Tent again to talk about what was changing, but her response was that everything was normal. A year later she had to take many months off work to cope with a nervous breakdown. As she emerged from that and many more months of resting, I wondered if it was more likely that her journey was nearly at an end. This is not to say that everyone has to have a very dramatic experience. The more recognition of the need to care for yourself in this transition, and the likelihood that life *will* change (also for the better!), the more accepting we can be.

I'm not yet travelling the menopause so I can only talk theoretically from the many women who've shared their experiences with me. Where there is a curiosity to engage with the inner work and acceptance that life will change, the fallout is likely to be less destabilising (or frightening), enabling the butterfly to emerge out of the cocoon more easily.

RESOURCES

Red School – Alexandra Pope and Sjanie Hugo-Wurlitzer run a fabulous weekend menopause workshop.

Jewels Wingfield – She also offers menopause workshops, including on sexuality and the menopause.

Commit to Kindness – Kate Codrington and Leora Leboff run a practice-based workshop called Love your Menopause.

Sue Monk Kidd and Ann Kidd Taylor (2011) *Travelling with Pomegranates*. Headline Review.

Bonnie Horrigan (1996) Red Moon Passage – *the Power and Wisdom of Menopause*. Harmony Books.

Susan Weed (2002) *New Menopausal Years: The Wise Woman Way*. Ash Tree Publishing.

Christiane Northrup (2012) *The Wisdom of Menopause: Creating Physical and Emotional Health during the Change.* Bantam Books.

Jane Lewis (2018) *Me and my Menopausal Vagina: Living with Vaginal Atrophy.* PAL books.

Concluding words

By now, rather than a necklace of pearls, I am visualising an intricate dreamcatcher with so many threads between the pearls. All the aspects that I have talked about separately are deeply connected and are critically important for creating a cocoon of safety.

What I have often found from the birth preparation workshops is that the techniques ripple out into other areas of life: work, parenting and life events. Much of the approach of this book can be applied to other experiences that you prepare for or encounter unexpectedly.

Reading through the book is a journey in itself, an initiation into birth wisdom and a transmission of women's knowledge from me to you.

I wish you well for your upcoming rite of passage. May you emerge empowered: a mother and a wiser woman.

Join other expectant mums at the Community of Pearls FB group to share your reflections and journey. A warm welcome awaits you there.

I look forward to hearing your birthing story.

Every baby's birth story has a heroine's journey woven into it.

Tessa

MOVE. BREATHE. RELAX. BE READY.

An online course to make what you've learnt in the book second nature in your body.

Would you like a range of practices organised in one place? To bring the book alive with pregnancy yoga and dance videos, breathing technique instruction, mindfulness and relaxation tracks (including hypnobirthing) and practical antenatal videos, visit www.pearlsofbirthwisdom.com.

Suitable throughout the second and third trimesters.

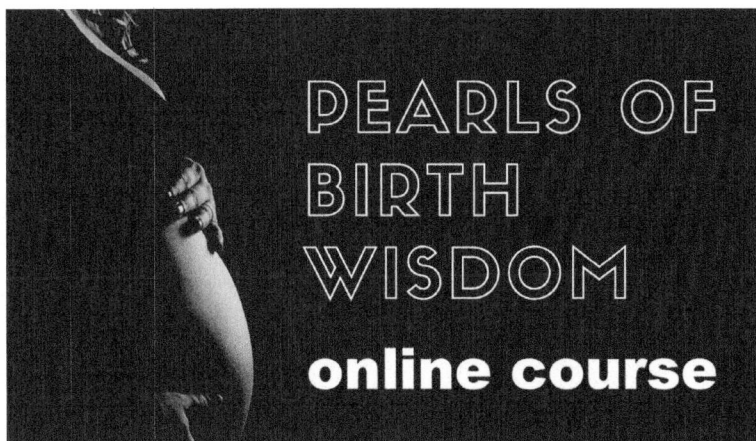

As a thank you for purchasing the book, you can get 25% off this affordable online course with coupon:

BOOK25off

(use on the check out page).

Tessa's other books:

The Pregnancy & Birth Colouring Book with Yoga Nidra:

Preparing for Birth throughMindfulness and Relaxation

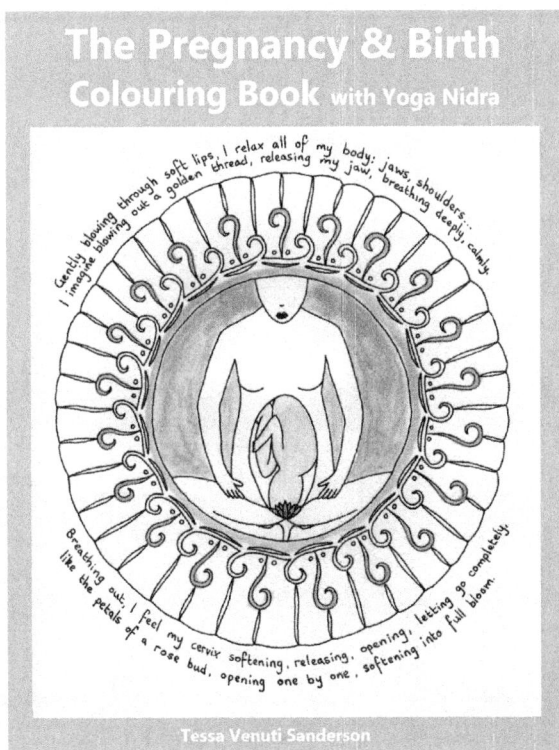

And three children's books around anatomy and puberty:

Ruby Luna's Curious Journey:
Follow Ruby Luna as she gets her period and transitions to secondary school

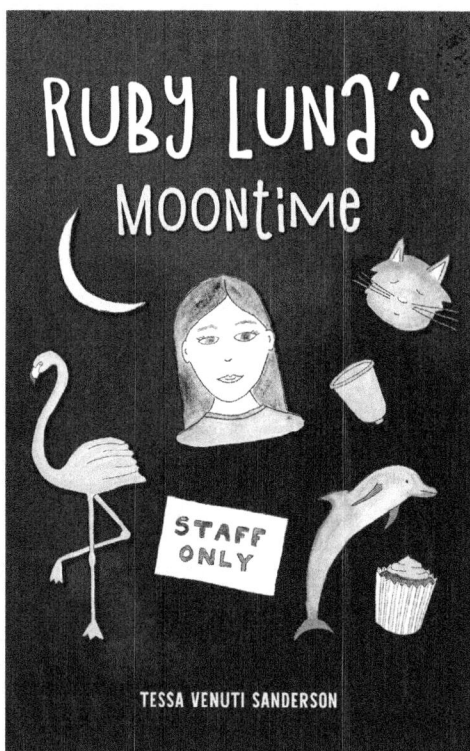

Ruby Luna's Curious Journey:

A girls' anatomy book covering puberty and periods

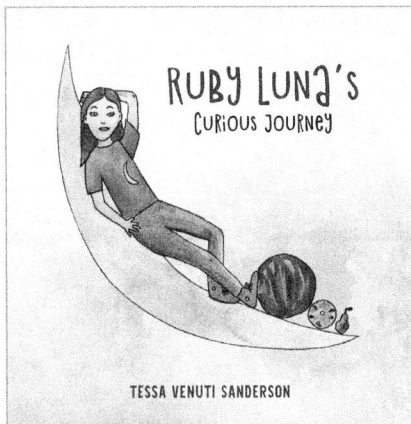

Dante Leon's Curious Journey:

A boys' illustrated anatomy and puberty book

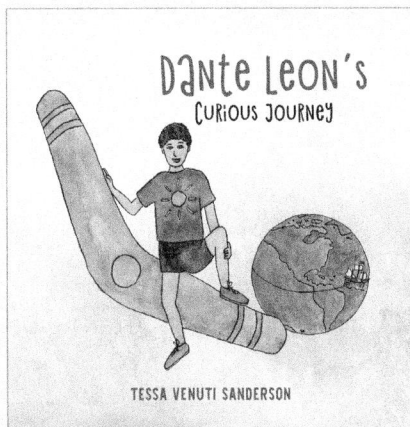

Printed in Great Britain
by Amazon